Contents

Foreword to the first edition

In Britain at least two million, probably more, old people have significant mental disorders, and in a huge country like the United States the numbers are even greater. Apart from their own suffering, there is that of relatives and others upon whom their illnesses impinge. And then there is the army of people in the health and social services – general practitioners, nurses, social workers, remedial staff, psychologists and many others – who become involved during the course of their work. More and more of them are making this work their special concern, as members of the teams which form the specialist old age psychiatry services which are now established in many areas. The pressing demand for education in this field is visible everywhere. Lectures and courses are usually oversubscribed, and participants ask for advice about what to read. This book will be high among those I shall be recommending.

When he came to join us in Nottingham, John Wattis was the first full-time university lecturer in the psychiatry of old age in Britain. He brought with him many talents: a flair for communication; and a gift both for getting on with people, and for getting on with the job. This ability to collaborate is reflected not only in the emphasis of this book, but in its successful joint authorship. Mike Church belongs to a profession the rich potential contribution of which to the field of geriatric psychiatry has still to be fully realised, and this book should give that process a boost.

A new introductory book to the rapidly growing field of old age psychiatry is welcome. There is sufficient detail and technical material here for intelligent people of all professions to get their teeth into, but it should not go beyond the understanding of any; and it presents well the many-sided practical and humane approach which is characteristic of its authors and of the developing speciality itself.

In the eight years since he came to work with us in Nottingham, John Wattis has become, through successive national surveys, the main recorder and archivist of our field. Having completed his training he moved on to start a service of his own in Leeds, an enterprise mounted in a time of economic difficulty, yet he has won golden opinions from all who know his work. He is Secretary of the Specialist Section on Old Age in the Royal College of Psychiatrists. That on top of all this he has found time to produce with his former colleague Mike Church this excellent little textbook, illustrates well his talent for getting on with things. Readers of this book will find themselves better informed, and infected with the authors' enthusiasm.

Tom Arie, MA BM FRCP FRCPsych FFCM,
Professor of Health Care of the Elderly,
University of Nottingham

Preface

The first edition of this book was suggested by Tom Arie, Professor of Health Care of the Elderly at the University of Nottingham. The seven years since the first edition of this book have seen a revolution in the way that Health Services in the United Kingdom are organized. One of the original co-authors, Mike Church, has moved on through several NHS posts to independent practice in the area of management consultancy. He has been replaced by Carol Martin, a lecturer in the Psychology of Old Age in our department.

In addition to the changes in the NHS there has been an explosion in the knowledge base of old age psychiatry, with several journals now devoted to the subject. A new diagnostic classificatory system (ICD10) has also been launched. In preparing this second edition, we have tried to remain true to the spirit of the first edition, whilst incorporating new knowledge and the changing context of our practice.

Throughout the text we have used the terms 'patient' and 'client' interchangeably. The people we serve are the same whatever we call them! We have also, generally, but not always referred to patients in the female gender, since this reflects the fact that more women than men survive into old age.

We have ordered the book so that the basic background information and skills in approaching the problems of old age are dealt with first. Then, using a problem-solving approach, we have dealt with the different symptoms that old people present to doctors, nurses, psychologists and others. Finally, we have dealt in more detail with approaches to management, stressing the importance of considering elderly patients as whole people interacting with their environments. We have sprinkled our account liberally with case-histories, as we believe this is the only way to do justice to the complexity of the situations faced in real life. At the same time, especially in preparing flow charts and other figures to summarise the work, we are aware that we have sometimes over-simplified. We have provided references for those who wish to pursue topics at greater depth.

We are indebted to our secretaries, and especially to the colleagues of all disciplines who have, in one way or another contributed to the development of the 2nd edition. Our thanks are also due to the journal *Geriatric Medicine* which has been proving ground for many of the ideas developed in this text. Our hope is that this book will provide an enjoyable and informative read, but at the same time that it will be a useful reference work for the busy practitioner, of whichever discipline.

1

Introduction

The last ten years have seen a change in views of ageing. *The Rising Tide* [1] is still rising, and certainly resources have been stretched, but there have also been changes in attitudes, legislation and the expectations of old people which make the issue of ageing more interesting than ever. A number of disciplines have now produced a significant body of research, which, if taken in by a wider society, might have profound implications for us all, even before we are old. Some of the ideas developed recently may well influence the demand for and provision of psychiatric services for old people. In this chapter, some of the basic facts and ideas about ageing and the elderly are presented in order to provide a context in which the provision of psychiatric services can be discussed.

1.1 WHAT IS 'OLD AGE'?

In the UK, there is a statutory retirement age for men at 65, which is the age at which people are legally defined as old in terms of public services such as pension rights and health. There is still some variability: the bus pass arrives at 60; working women remain unsure whether they are to retire at 60 or 65; some health services for old people are restricted to the very old (70 or 75), but most use 65 as the cut-off. However, this number is somewhat arbitrary. Old and young are comparative terms, and individuals, including advertisers, change their opinion on when old age starts. It is a significant point, for example, when we realize that we have passed an age when we had dismissed someone as old – such as 30 – and find that we ourselves do not feel 'past it'! Perhaps a better question to ask than 'When am I old?' is 'When am I too old for what?' For everybody, getting older is an issue even from childhood, as it seems clear then that birthdays bring advantage and privileges.

Concerns about ageing, however, start early in adulthood, with worries over reaching the milestones we have planned. For example, ageing becomes a prominent issue for some women in their twenties and thirties when they struggle over the juggling act of relationships, career and children. Most people take active notice of the process of physical ageing by this point in their lives, and mid-life is an accepted point for review, if not crisis.

It is possible to measure age along a number of dimensions. There is, of course, chronological age. In addition, it is worth considering biological age, which overlaps with fitness and health; psychological age, related to level of intellectual maturity and psycho-social development; perceived age, which may contain elements of how old the person feels and is seen to be; and social age, related to position in terms of career or family milestones, for example. An individual may well be at different stages in all these [2].

People have the potential for development throughout their lives. Development is a dynamic process, and occurs when an individual has to face a new situation and to learn new skills, resolve internal conflicts or take on a new role. Some of these are the normal transitions of life, such as retirement; others are idiosyncratic changes, such as disability, divorce or the loss of a child. The human potential for creative solutions to dilemmas and problems leads to a wide variation in skills, lifestyles and coping strategies by the time people grow old.

1.2 NORMAL AGEING AND ADAPTATION TO CHANGE

In addition to the potential for varied solutions to life's problems, there are some changes that occur predictably and can be considered a normal part of ageing. In the area of cognition, for example, research suggests normal trends with ageing. Response time slows; that is, it takes longer for older people to process new information. The actual size of the change is small (less than a half of a second in most research) but in some circumstances even that may be critical, especially in combination with sensory or motor changes or stress. Many older people can compensate by developing skills and strategies. For example, older typists look further ahead when typing and have extra time for processing, thereby maintaining speed.

Even minor illness may have important effects on cognitive functioning. Speed of information-processing is related to age, but retrieval of memories or information may, however, be related in part to mental health. Some suggest that old people trade speed for accuracy, and indeed, expertise does not decline with age, even though new skills less easily become automatic. The differences found are statistical ones between groups and there are older individuals whose performance matches or exceeds that of younger ones. Training older people to use their memories and asking them to perform in areas of special competence allows them to perform as well as younger ones. Factors such as depression and dementia affect memory; so does inactivity, lack of motivation or boredom. Memories for events in the distant past are not necessarily better than memory for recent events; some of the stories retained by individuals may be overlearned and told in an automatic, repetitive way. In normal ageing, it seems that the ordinary tasks involving memory, such as sending someone a birthday card or remembering that the bath is running, do not decline with age. Where motivation is high, older people may be better at telephoning someone at a set time, for example, but apparently perform less well when tasks are not seen as vital. Certainly, older people have a tendency to complain that they are more forgetful, particularly of names and the last place in which they put something. There is a suggestion that the thinking of old people becomes more context-bound, more expertise-related, and intuitive because it is more efficient to proceed in this way. The disadvantage would be a greater risk of difficulty adapting in a new environment. For more detail, the reader might turn to texts on ageing [2, 3]. Old people are often thought to develop wisdom. Wisdom can be defined as a capacity to exercise good judgement when important issues are complex and uncertain. Wisdom requires the integration of thought and emotion, and reflexivity, in order to take into account ambiguity and context, and wise people allow for there to be a number of possible solutions to a problem [4].

As regards personality, there is research evidence for the importance of both change and continuity throughout adult life. While people's characters tend to remain stable over long periods, stressful life events may require adaptations and promote change. In particular, it seems that some events, such as separation by divorce or bereavement, may set in motion a series of changes and decision-making with long-term and profound effects. However, personality types seem to remain stable throughout adult life, while the level of life satisfaction is related to personality type rather than age. Some researchers have sought to identify common strategies for dealing with ageing itself. One such strand is the reclaiming of opposite-gender characteristics [5]. Adaptation to stress is important to life satisfaction. Older people tend to see stress in a wider context, so are sometimes less bothered by minor stresses. In old age, changes are often forced on the lifestyle of the person by events such as disability or bereavement. One change often precipitates others; for example, the death of a spouse may necessitate moving from the marital home. A stable relationship with a confidant offers important protection to morale and mental stability, although it cannot always outweigh the effects of, for example, physical illness.

1.3 SOME FACTS ON AGEING

Most books on old age start with a section on the demography of ageing. This one is no exception. The increase in the proportion and numbers of old people in the population is worldwide, and is at least as marked in the Third World as anywhere. In less than ten years, it is estimated that there will be about 600 million people over 60 alive, and about two-thirds will be living in Third World countries. This country now counts (or discounts, if you prefer) one in six of its population as elderly. This adds up to over eight million individuals over 65 years of age, of whom about three-quarters of a million are over 85 years old (see Table 1.1). The role of this group is therefore likely to have important implications for the whole of the population [6]. The increase in numbers of old people has been due to improvements in public health, reductions of child deaths and increased quality of life. However, as the number of old people increases, so does the number of very old people (to 800 000 in total over 85 years in Britain in 1991) suffering from either dementia (to one in five) or a chronic illness which compromises independent living (to three in five) [6, 7].

Table 1.1 Estimates of the number of old people in Great Britain

Census date	*Total population* (millions)	*Age Group* 65–74	75–84	85+	*Age* 65+	75+	85+
		(population in millions)			(% of total population)		
1981	54.3	5.0	2.6	0.6	15.1	5.9	1.1
1991	55.4	5.0	3.0	0.8	15.9	6.9	1.4
2001 (predicted)	56.4	4.6	3.0	1.0	15.2	7.1	1.8

Further, the gender ratio of this group is skewed. For those alive now, there is an increase in the ratio of women to men from around 50 years of age, until at age 65 there are over 120 women to 100 men. At age 95 and above there are about five times as many women alive as men. This too has implications for the possible contributions and needs of old people. At the most concrete end of the spectrum, the financial resources of women have always been lower than those of men. They earn less when they work, so have less at retirement. Old people as a group are more likely to live in sub-standard accommodation. The gender gap has implications in its turn for domestic arrangements. Women have tended to marry older men, and survive longer. A significant proportion of old people, mostly women, live alone. Over 80 per cent of women over 75 years are single, divorced or widowed. Services for very old people are, in the main, services for women. Women have been relatively excluded from public life, and the current cohorts of old women include fewer highly educated and professional people than their male peer group or younger women. For women, a proportion of their influence and desirability is determined by looks, and cultural views of a beautiful woman mean a young woman. Many older women were brought up with an ideal of woman as passive or receptive, restricted and punished if they showed signs of asserting themselves. This suggests that old people may be restricted in their ability as a group to exert a wider influence. This is an example of the cohort effect;

younger women have more access to education, careers and a range of role models, which affect their expectations and behaviour currently and will continue to do so into old age [8].

In terms of knowledge and expertise, it is likely that old people will be excluded as the need for their skills, gained in an industrial society, seems to reduce; further, women have had less access to the professions, managerial posts and skilled work in their working life. (Just occasionally, the loss of old people at retirement is seen to be problematic; recently, British Rail found that its younger employees had no knowledge of particular procedures.) Old people have less access to (and can feel undeserving of) even basic education after retirement, and are likely to struggle with innovations such as computers, even though they have the potential for learning the necessary skills. Overall, the result has to be a disenfranchisement of old people in social, cultural and political spheres. Decisions on public spending and service priority, including those influencing provisions for old people, are made by people under retirement age, even if the views of the retired are researched and taken into account.

There is a common view that the increase in old people means an increase in the total burden for the working population. This appears to be a fallacy in developed countries, where the number of children is reduced and the age profile of the population is more even. Coleman and Bond [6] argue that age is unlikely to be the most important factor for change in post-industrial society. Given the changes in health and resources of old people, perhaps the task for developed countries is to allow for a greater flexibility in the opportunities and services open to the old, enabling them to play a greater part. Currently, however, in Britain at least, old people lose their social position and can be isolated and lonely. Families are now smaller, communities less stable, divorce more common, and there are both fewer younger women relative to the number of old people and fewer women who are not in paid employment. All these changes mean that the contribution of old people may have to be made outside their immediate family, and that care will be less likely to be provided by the family.

These considerations directly affect psychiatric services for old people. Increasingly, there will be a need for support for old people suffering from dementia that cannot be supplied by the family. With increasing living standards and expectations among the population as a whole, there may in future be higher levels of stress and dissatisfaction among some groups of old people regarding their life circumstances, which may on occasion lead to mental illness. Individuals may more actively struggle with changes in self-esteem as they face the disturbing and demoralizing images that they and others have of themselves as old people. There may be a greater demand for psychological services and counselling, as a cohort of old people brought up post-Freud struggle to achieve a satisfactory adaptation in late life in a situation where there are few acceptable, and fewer desirable, role models. Increasingly, old people may feel entitled to more choice and autonomy, and to affect the type of services provided.

In general, old people have fewer resources than other adults and are under-used by the society within which we live. There is a risk that the situation remains static as the elderly, being an economically unproductive group, are not provided with the necessary resources to remedy their situation, because they would be wasted. The rationale is, 'They will be dead soon, anyway.' Old people themselves, having been brought up with this view, do not always see how it might be to the advantage of younger people as well as themselves if they were to take a more active part in, for example, community activities and politics. Images of retirement range from 'permanent holiday well-deserved after a lifetime of sometimes unsatisfying paid work' to 'burden on the working population'.

1.4 IMAGES OF AGEING AND AGEISM

Images of old age have a continuity across recent history and Western culture. Featherstone and Hepworth [9] have described images of ageing as they have changed over the centuries and point out that there is a balance between the value accorded to young and old, which shifted towards youth with the post-war baby boom, and may return as that cohort ages. They describe the current limits of middle age as 'mid-thirties to late sixties'. Whatever the particular images of old age, each contains an implicit comparison with youth, so that people are approved for ageing well (looking young), or castigated for impersonating youth (mutton dressed as lamb). They note the creation of positive images of several types as the old are developed as a consumer group. Commonly, there are images of the youthful old person, linked to anti-ageing products, and the image of retirement as a leisure lifestyle, linked to leisure goods and activities. While these may raise the consciousness of both old and young, the risk would be in increased dissatisfaction among those who see opportunities but cannot attain them.

Ageism is the expression of disadvantage due to age and is noticeable everywhere, psychiatric services not excepted! Like sexism, it is often invisible and is highly reinforced. It is built into the social networks and institutions in which we work and live, and its effects start in youth. In Britain, as in many other societies, images of beauty and goodness are associated with youth. Our definitions of old age are bound up with our views of other phenomena, including infirmity, dependency, aesthetics, moral and social ideals, gender attributes, independence, competence and employment. Culturally, younger people play a significant role in the definitions and experience of ageing. The healthy under-sixty-fives write the soaps and the newspapers, deliver conference papers, treat old people in hospital and serve to them in shops!

To describe someone as old is often seen as abusive. One young man, introducing his mother and grandmother to a friend, innocently said, 'Guess which is which!' If his friend could not tell beforehand, he definitely could afterwards. The idea of old age as a handicap remains prevalent even among trained psychiatric staff. In a teaching exercise, one of the authors routinely asked nurses to think of and describe an old person known personally to them. In each session, virtually everyone who described someone old in positive terms agreed that they thought the individual was exceptional for their age.

1.5 DEVELOPMENT INTO OLD AGE

The majority of people have a rough plan for their lives; in our culture, perhaps in all, they want partners and families, friendship, productive and interesting work and leisure activities. These plans are laid down in childhood along with the characteristics and skills that may enable them to realize their potential. Fairy tales may owe some of their popularity to the reassurance they offer to children that they may realize adult goals. Some people's lives approach their desired life plan; others do not. The degree of satisfaction with life in earlier stages, and the decisions made, have important implications for later opportunities and experiences. For example, most people marry or have long-standing partnerships during the early years of adulthood. The social norm and the desirable outcome (at least as far as parents go) is marriage and a family.

Mid-life is often a time for reconsidering the structure and aims of life, and while for some people there is relatively little sign of a mid-life crisis, others may make major changes. While it is increasingly the case that variations of this theme are accepted, and may prove satisfactory, there are some life strategies with profound implications for old age. For example, a woman who puts off marriage and child-bearing until later in life may find it harder to achieve these aims. She may succeed in making a traditional marriage, but also might have a child alone, or remain happily or unhappily childless. This leads to one of the main criticisms of the use of developmental theory in late life: that, by virtue of different capacities, interests, decisions and opportunities, there is more variety than uniformity. This may be so, although even in terms of superficial interests and opinions, themes are often apparent.

At a deeper level, however, there do seem to be issues common to people of particular ages and generations. Erikson [10, 11] suggested that a dominant conflict for old people is that of 'integrity versus despair', as they struggle to come to terms with the limits of their existence, their achievements and the loss of a future. Erikson's model is based on psychoanalytic theory, and implies that personal growth is achieved through the successful resolution of psycho-social conflicts which are brought about by maturational processes and external conditions. A number of others have used psychoanalytic theory to understand or explain themes that occur during later life.

Gutmann [5] studied the older people in three societies using a primarily qualitative methodology, and compared themes from interviews across all three to minimize the effects of local beliefs and specific cultural conditions. The themes emerging for men included those of physical comfort and especially food (orality), and for women there was a frequent pattern of increased assertiveness. Gutmann provides a model of this process with what he calls the 'sexual diamond'. Given that there are pressures and limits on the achievement of psycho-social tasks, for example, employment and educational opportunities are different for men and women, many people allocate tasks or qualities according to gender. Women are supposed to be nurturing and communicative, men to be strong, assertive and protective. Because of social conditions and expectations, those who do not follow the conventional pattern may well experience more difficulties and stress. This is in line with clinical experience; in one study of psychodynamic psychotherapy, young men tended to express concern about mastery and competition, while older men were more likely to deal with dependency needs [12].

Gilligan [13] suggested that Erikson's model, like other research, is limited in its usefulness, describing the developmental path of men not women. She suggested that women continually negotiate a balance between autonomy and relationship. The model probably only holds for a proportion of men in cultures which have this life course as the ideal. In Japanese culture, for example, individuality is stressed less than collective effort. People have many different strands to their life and may deal more successfully with some areas than others. Nemiroff and Colarusso [14] have proposed ten major themes which play a part throughout adult life into old age, which are outlined in Table 1.2 and exemplified in Table 1.3.

Erikson's model suggests that all the conflicts he defines are being continually renegotiated. For example, if in adult life, someone is betrayed by a partner, the balance of trust may be changed towards mistrust. The degree of the change and its permanence will be dependent on past experiences. If the person's own background was stable and loving, this may allow for the repair of the relationship or reinvestment in another. If, on the other hand, the person had been severely let down or abused by a parent, it might be difficult or impossible to overcome the adult trauma constructively. A supportive family or friends may help; so may therapy. If not overcome, such mistrust may be increasingly important in old age as the person faces reductions in strength and independence while fearing that carers will behave in an untrustworthy fashion.

This theory may go some way to explain the occurrence of distress and severe symptomatology in late life. If in adult

Table 1.2 Adult developmental lines

1. love, sex and intimacy
2. the body
3. time and death
4. relationship to children
5. relationship to parents
6. mentor relationship
7. relationship to society
8. work
9. play
10. finances

Source: Nemiroff and Colarusso [14]

life people avoid developing skills to cope with problematic issues, necessary for intimate relationships and dependency, or in order to act autonomously without excessive anxiety, then the changes brought about by ageing, such as frailty or bereavement, may sometimes bring them face to face with the problem and their failure [15].

1.6 THE CHALLENGES OF OLD AGE

There are several issues common to old people regardless of culture, gender, or education. This is not to say that these factors have no effect on the experience of old age; indeed, they have profound implications for the resources and health of old people and the beliefs, held both by old people themselves and those not yet old, about ageing. Some of these are summarized in Table 1.3.

1.6.1 The body

Bodily changes are basic to ageing, and these changes can affect psychological functioning. With improvements in lifestyle and diet, old people can generally remain fit and well. Many of the impairments of old age are the effects of chronic illness, lack of exercise and poor diet. For example, the extent of osteoporosis can be reduced by exercise, diet and hormones. The prevention of this disease might have not only an effect on mobility and the rate of fractures in older women, but have effects on levels of depression and self-esteem. The effect of changes in ap-

Table 1.3 The issues of old age

Maintaining close relationships with others
Looking after sexual needs
Using time well and maintaining meaningful activity
Using material resources well
Bodily change; disability
Death of self and others
Transitions; retirement, grand parenthood
Dealing with images of old age and oneself as old
Changes in control and autonomy

pearance should not be under-estimated. A proportion of old people cannot accept the change in their looks or strength with equanimity. It signals a loss in social and sexual status for which they can find no compensation, yet it is seen as shameful to mind. The importance of physical change has been underlined in popular literature by Germaine Greer, who has explored the meaning of Hormone Replacement Therapy for menopausal women. She suggests that HRT is offered in part as a 'cure' for ageing [16]. Although some people may celebrate their wrinkles, it is often part of therapeutic work with old people to help them as they struggle to come to terms with the impact of physical changes on their activities, relationships, self-esteem and mood.

Expectations about health have an important part to play in old people's satisfaction. For example, a recent study suggested that older people describe themselves as sufficiently fit if they can carry out the tasks of daily living, even though these may require minimal activity. Levels of fitness in the general population may be much lower than optimal and many people may be accepting restrictions on their lifestyle unnecessarily [17].

1.6.2 Transitions and stress

The passage into old age requires an individual to adapt to a number of transitions. These include both normal changes, such as retirement or having grandchildren, and idiosyncratic ones, such as taking an educational course post-retirement, bereavement or late divorce. Many old people do adapt well to these changes, whether they are crises or not. Others may have difficulties even with the predictable events. Sometimes it is possible to see how the problems have arisen in retrospect. For example, a man who has difficulties with intimate relationships but remains happily bound up with his work may retire to find that he and his wife have different expectations. If the couple cannot come to a satisfactory resolution, it is possible that one might present with symptoms of depression, anxiety or somatic complaints (see Case 8.6). Psychiatric services might in this case be called in to offer help in negotiating the transition. Bereavement counselling, groups for individuals suffering from isolation or interpersonal difficulties, family therapy and individual therapy may all be helpful to individuals coping with transitions.

One of the psychological tasks of old age is that of maintaining self-esteem in the face of the negative images we all carry of ageing. The success with which an individual may achieve this task is related to earlier experiences of self-acceptance. When this goes well, the old person will have developed sufficient confidence in order to adapt in a flexible and assertive manner. Without this confidence, individuals may resist changes even if this means suffering isolation or loss. An example might be the person who refuses a hearing-aid or a Day Centre place because it would be felt to be humiliating. One of the tasks facing the professionals in psychiatric services for old people is that of helping vulnerable people to accept help which in no way makes up for what has been lost, but can make adaptation possible.

1.6.3 Control and autonomy; power

Some of the changes in old age make it more difficult for people to exercise choice or control over their lives, or even themselves. Physical changes, institutional settings, dementia and restrictive beliefs can all have this effect, often impairing an old person's mental health. While sometimes it is impossible to proceed without reducing a person's choice, it is an important task within the psychiatric services for old people to attempt to reverse this trend, enabling old people to decide on their own lifestyle as much as is possible. Langer [18] showed that there were differences in several psychological dimensions and even rates of mortality between a group of old people in institutional care encouraged to take responsibility for their own lives and a group encouraged to look to staff for the satisfaction of their needs.

For some old people, self-determination is limited by factors other than ageing. Gender, racial and cultural influences operate throughout life and the resources and influence accrued over the years can buffer some of the effects of ageing. A small group of wealthy older women control a large proportion of privately owned wealth in the United States, often through having survived their husbands. Senior positions in the professions and important social and political positions are occupied by older people.

As well as material constraints, there are psychological ones. Not only is there the view that old age is a time for leisure rather than active involvement in social and familial activities, but many experience anxieties about helplessness [19]. When these anxieties trouble the person, it may lead to inappropriate attempts at avoidance or control.

1.6.4 Sexuality

Pearl King [20], in her description of the problems of bringing older people into therapy in late life, lists concerns over sexuality as a major theme. She comments that the resolution of these issues revives conflicts similar to those of adolescence. The middle-aged man who leaves his wife for a younger woman provides a commonplace example of the use of sexuality in the maintenance of self-esteem (a man who has an attractive woman being more highly regarded) and protection against anxieties (of failing powers and infirmity or eventual death). The American television series 'The Golden Girls' provides another; they behave as teenagers might, being concerned with relationships and their looks. For women, sexuality in old age is affected not only by beliefs, but is pre-dated by the menopause. Older women, perhaps unsurprisingly, see the menopause more favourably than younger ones, and do not view it as a major transition. For both men and women, there are some changes in sexual response, but not of an order that precludes sexual activity. Contrary to the opinion of younger people, many individuals and couples continue sexual relations into their seventies or longer. In most heterosexual couples who give up sexual activity, it is stopped by the male partner. One of the authors has successfully treated a number of older men suffering from sexual difficulties. For many women, there are difficulties in maintaining sexual activity, partly because of the proportion who live without partners. Again, it has proved useful for some of these to have had the opportunity to talk about their situation, and to consider the options open to them [21]. Unfortunately, however, the choices remain limited, partly because older men are often concerned to find younger partners. Some women, it must be said, welcome the freedom that living alone brings, and avoid relationships in case they are restricted or are required to provide care for an older man.

1.6.5 Death and bereavement

Old age requires people to face death. It is in late adulthood especially that individuals have to come to terms with the meaning of their existence and decide for themselves if their life has been worthwhile. This experience can be seen in Erikson's last stage, described as 'Integrity versus Despair' [10]. This is often presaged by an increased awareness of time limits and reduced opportunities. From the successful resolution of this evaluation emerges the traditional quality attributed to old age: wisdom. Fear of death seems to become less common as people age [22]. This is partly perhaps because of having survived frightening or stressful events in life by which the experience of death can be estimated. However, preparation for death, for example, leaving a will, is relatively uncommon, perhaps indicating a more or less healthy denial.

Kubler-Ross [23] has described a series of reactions that individuals tend to experience if faced with the prospect of their own death. These include: denial of death and isolation from others through difficulty in communicating meaningfully; depression and despair; anger; attempts to bargain and control; acceptance and hope. It is difficult to predict which feelings individuals may experience, or in what order [23].

Many old people find their time can still be meaningful, but a common clinical problem is that of the demoralized and desperate old person, who seems to feel that life is already over or is passing them by. They have difficulty in finding a reason to carry on or any meaning to their experience. Retirement, losses and discontinuities can lead up to such states of mind. Bereavement can be a cause of such feelings for some. The impact of bereavement should not be under-estimated in old age even though it is almost an inevitable crisis [24]. The meaning of loss through death can be varied and the mourning process will be greatly affected by this. For example, loss of a spouse may bring about loss of a companion, loss or change in material resources and conditions or even changes in self-definition. Beliefs about oneself may be important in surviving a loss. For example, if a person believes they cannot cope without their partner or that it is awful to be old and alone, there may seem no incentive to make new contacts or even to take on the household tasks previously done by the other person. People complain more to their doctors, and there is increased risk of mortality, after a bereavement. Models of grieving, like those of facing one's own death, are conceptualized as stages. The perception of loss has to take place first, and is followed by protest or search, despair and grief, then evolves into detachment from the lost person and reinvestment in other relationships or activities. These models simplify the reality of a person's experience. Rather, it seems that individuals reiterate their grief with each reminder of their loss. Some individuals find their loss so painful that they protect themselves from grief in a variety of ways, leading to prolonged states of depression or unconstructive action.

On the other hand, older adults are increasingly interested in psychological therapies including psychoanalysis. Pearl King, from her experience of work with older adults, has talked about the possible advantages of working with older people [25]. These include an awareness of the pressure of time, which can increase motivation; stability, and increased financial resources compared to younger adults. She has recognized that a group of adults seek psychotherapy as they approach old age. They are concerned to make the best of their later years, after perhaps recognizing the emptiness inside themselves, the failures they have experienced in developing their potential, or the difficulties they have in relationships. Such people wish for therapy to help them make the best of the time and resources available to them and use therapy well.

Freud thought that old people would not benefit from psychoanalysis, but recently, the work of both clinicians and academics has added to our understanding of ageing. Kathleen Woodward [26] has examined the limits placed on Freud's thought not just by culture (after all, the threat of social disapprobation did not stop him theorizing about sex, dreams or the unconscious), but by his own conflicts. She makes explicit links between Freud's publications and his personal concerns as expressed in his letters, and explores the way he could not recognize his own ageism because of his fears of ageing and unresolved feelings about family relationships. She goes on to use examples from literature to show how people approach the old, ageing and death in different ways, and suggests that our understanding of these can be enriched through psychoanalytic theory [26]. This work, and literature itself, can add depth and richness to our understanding of our patients' experience.

1.7 IMPLICATIONS FOR SERVICES

The previous sections contain material which has important implications when thinking of psychiatric services for old people. For example, it points up the difficulties in defining a service or the target population by a birth date alone, because the potential problems brought by patients are so varied. It is also clear that expectations and beliefs about what is normal, desirable or pathological in terms of age may affect the nature and usefulness of a service. The philosophy of ageing held by the developers, purchasers and providers of a service, whether held explicitly or implicitly embedded within decision-making or planning processes, will affect its priorities, aims and the range of treatments offered. However, beliefs and attitudes can be discussed and revised in the light of evidence. Those working in psychiatric services for old people need then to take into account their own ideas and definitions of ageing. Often, we, like others, may be satisfied with too little, because, 'after all, what else can you expect at this age?' Research on normal ageing, for example on the nature and extent of cognitive change in late life, and on the life cycle, can give a more optimistic view of the potentials of old people.

For many old people, their use of the services may be relatively straightforward. Physical illness and psychiatric conditions can be diagnosed, some conditions treated successfully, others like dementia, managed. Even this requires a specialized knowledge of ageing, and of the issues relevant to coping with disability. These issues may be similar for people of all ages, but old people have to face a different set of implications and life circumstances. For example, when a man's wife dies at thirty, he will have to deal with an event that is unusual and unexpected among his peers, but he may have more opportunity to remarry than a man whose wife dies when he is 70, even though this is a more 'normal' event. Under these circumstances, the young man might grieve and then seek a new partner, while the older man might have to adapt to living alone and satisfying his emotional needs through friendships and family. If referred for depression to a service, both might benefit from a range of approaches, from anti-depressants, to bereavement counselling, or social skills training. The older man will probably be provided with help in the home and day care, yet his problem is likely to be only partially practical. It is important to consider why both he and service providers consider practical support satisfactory, as opposed, say, to developing new skills, both practical (so he can run his own household and maybe develop an interest in cooking) and psychological (to be able to identify his needs for companionship and set about satisfying them).

Old people have as much capacity to enjoy life as young ones, and many do, adapting to the changes they have to face; but some do not. Often, failure to adapt results from difficulty facing loss, sometimes of people, sometimes of resources, sometimes of role, but perhaps always loss of meaning, which is necessary to make life satisfying. In addition to any medical or physical interventions, services for old people have to take into account the impact of this loss of earlier satisfaction, and help old people in their attempt to recreate meaning and satisfactory lives. This includes the need to recognize attempts that cause problems for themselves or others, such as the use of physical illness to gain the contact they feel is necessary.

Recognition does not, of course, mean that we can then always provide a cure, but this holds true for all age groups. Older people more often face difficulties that cannot be changed, such as poverty and physical disability. There are many instances when we have to work with old people who are in pain or distressed, and there is nothing to be done to stop this. This makes the work distressing at times for the professionals. If not supported and helped to understand clinical situations, staff can end up discouraged and liable to avoid the patient's pain. For this reason, staff support and good training are essential parts of any service.

Over the last few years, there have also been structural changes to which services are having to adapt. These include changes to community facilities, and notably an increase in voluntary and (mostly) private sector residential and nursing home provision. In some services, given the available resources and concern about the disorientating effect of unnecessary moves on demented patients, the NHS no longer offers intermittent care on a regular basis. Day-hospital places have become an increasingly important resource for assessment, treatment and follow-up and in some areas operate as the focus for the service, acting as a front-line between community and hospital admission. With the development of individual treatment plans, they offer far more than a necessary break for a carer. The day hospital does offer a social environment for an isolated and depressed individual, for example, but is also likely to be aiming at the development of a new network of social support on discharge, or the improvement of social skills within its relatively protected setting.

Currently, changes in the status of NHS services as they are re-organized into Trusts have implications for the links between services. The full potential for General Practitioners to affect the shape of services has not yet been experienced. Internal 'market forces' have yet to operate. These changes signal a different view of the patient, and a different role for staff offering services or choosing them for their patients, aiming to give patients more choice. On the other hand, funding and contractual arrangements may make it difficult to access particular resources. Mentally ill old people are often unable to protest effectively and in the absence of advocacy may suffer unnecessary hardship. At present, there has been relatively little chance to explore and integrate the views of old people into the planning of services. It is difficult to envisage the changes that increased flexibility and consumer choice might bring over the coming years, but it seems unlikely that old people would choose the current situation. A number of the authors' concerns are mentioned below.

The transfer of the bulk of residential and nursing care to the private sector gives cause for concern. While there are regulations about the quality of care, staffing and training in private sector institutions, their access to and use of occupational therapy, physiotherapy and psychological services may be restricted. Regulations may be hard to enforce where there are concerns about the quality of care, especially when it is the psychological aspect of an institution that causes anxiety.

Most Homes operate on a nursing or hotel model, where control is very firmly in the hands of the staff, not the residents. Often the Home is owned by the senior staff, but no core training is available or required. Residents may have little choice over the routines and conditions under which they live and may under some circumstances find they have no rights to stay in a Home, nor find it possible to leave if they are unhappy. Although many Homes are run by sensitive and caring people, the aim of self-determination is rarely high on the list of priorities. The implications of research findings such as that of Langer need careful consideration, given the suggestion that mobility, mental well-being and even mortality are affected by the milieu in which an old person lives [18].

One aspect of service provision that may significantly benefit the quality of life of the old person facing difficulties is access to counselling and advice before major decisions, such as moving house after bereavement, are made. When an old person is distressed, referral to psychological services may enable some people to adapt to change without becoming seriously disturbed, while hospital and medical provision become necessary only for those individuals who are unable or unwilling to use these. The group of patients described in a derogatory way as the 'worried well' (and which is comprised of distressed and anxious people who are finding it difficult to cope) may benefit from such an opportunity, thereby facilitating better adaptation. Elderly people have until recently been reluctant to use specialist psychiatric services because of the images of senility and dependence associated with them. With the limited resources available, this may be just as well. In the future, they may also be put off by others from using the service because they are not old and ill enough. It is easy to envisage a situation where a proportion of the population who are demoralized or distressed, has effectively no access to psychiatric or psychological services because they are too old for adult services and not impaired enough by dementia, suicidal feelings or psychosis to be referred to the services provided for old people.

On the other hand, changes in the ways in which ageing is seen may lead to an increase in the expectations of older people, so that they both look after their health better, feel more able to influence the communities in which they live, and assert themselves more. Under such circumstances, they themselves may let service providers know more clearly what they need.

REFERENCES

1. National Health Service, Health Advisory Service (1982) *The Rising Tide: Developing Services for Mental Illness in Old Age*, NHS Health Advisory Service, Sutton, Surrey.
2. Kimmel, D. (1990) *Adulthood and Aging*, Wiley, London.
3. Bond, J. and Coleman, P. (eds) (1990) *Ageing in Society: an Introduction to Social Gerontology*, Sage, London.
4. Woods, R.T. and Britton, P.G. (1985) *Clinical Psychology with the Elderly*, Croom Helm, London.
5. Gutmann, D. (1987) *Reclaimed Powers: Towards a New Psychology of Men and Women in Later Life*, Basic Books, New York.
6. Coleman, P. and Bond, J. (1990) Ageing in the twentieth century, in *Ageing in Society: an Introduction to Social Gerontology*, (eds J. Bond and P. Coleman), Sage, London.
7. Keen, J. (1992) *Dementia*, Office of Health Economics, London.
8. Bardwick, J.M. (1990) Who we are and what we want: a psychological model, in *New Dimensions in Adult Development*, (eds R.A. Nemiroff and C.A. Colarusso), Basic Books, New York.
9. Featherstone, M. and Hepworth, M. (1990) Images of ageing, in *Ageing in Society: an Introduction to Social Gerontology*, (eds J. Bond and P. Coleman), Sage, London.
10. Erikson, E.H. (1965) *Childhood and Society*, Norton, New York.
11. Erikson, E.H., Erikson, J.M. and Kivnick, H.Q. (1986) *Vital Involvement in Old Age: the Experience of Old Age in Our Time*, Norton, New York.
12. Hildebrand, H.P. (1986) Psychodynamic psychotherapy with the elderly, in *Psychological Therapies for the Elderly*, (eds I. Hanley and M. Gilhooly), Croom Helm, London.
13. Gilligan, C. (1982) *In a Different Voice: Psychological Theory and Women's Development*, Harvard University Press, Cambridge, MA.
14. Nemiroff, R.A. and Colarusso, C.A. (1980) *Adult Development*, Basic Books, New York.
15. Jacobwitz, J. and Newton, N. (1990) Time, context and character: a

lifespan view of psychopathology during the second half of life, in *New Dimensions in Adult Development*, (eds R.A. Nemiroff and C.A. Colarusso), Basic Books, New York.
16. Greer, G. (1992) *The Change*, Penguin Books, Harmondsworth.
17. Briggs, R. (1990) Biological ageing, in *Ageing in Society: an Introduction to Social Gerontology*, (eds J. Bond and P. Coleman), Sage, London.
18. Langer, E.J. (1983) *The Psychology of Control*, Sage, Beverley Hills, California.
19. Martindale, B. (1989) Becoming dependent again: the fears of some elderly persons and a younger therapist. *Psychoanalytic Psychotherapy*, **4**, 67–75.
20. King, P.H. (1980) The lifecycle as indicated by the transference in the psychoanalysis of the middle-aged and elderly. *International Journal of Psycho-Analysis*, **61**, 153–60.
21. Martin, C. (1992) The elder and the other, *Free Associations*, **27**, 341–54.
22. Bengston, V.L., Cuellar, J.B. and Ragan, P.K. (1977) Stratum contrasts and similarities in attitudes towards death. *Journal of Gerontology*, **32**, 76–88.
23. Kubler-Ross, E. (1969) *On Death and Dying*, Macmillan, New York.
24. Dershimer, R. (1990) *Counselling the Bereaved*, Psychology Practitioner Handbooks, Pergamon Press, Oxford.
25. King, P. (1992) *The Challenge*. Lecture given at The Institute of Psycho-Analysis, London.
26. Woodward, K. (1991) *Ageing and its Discontents: Freud and Other Fictions*, Indiana University Press, Indianapolis.

2

Assessment

The skills needed to assess and formulate the management of elderly patients are best developed in supervised clinical practice including review of outcome in individual patients. The self-discipline of careful assessment, problem formulation and review of outcome is the foundation for professional growth. This chapter will deal with the psychiatric and psychological assessment of older people as a framework for such learning. Physical, social and other forms of assessment will also be covered briefly. The self-discipline of good practice in record-keeping and review can be improved by the practice of regular peer-group audit which, like self-assessment depends on careful record-keeping. Assessment of the patient is not a 'one-off' phenomenon. It needs to be repeated throughout treatment in order to evaluate progress and, if necessary, modify treatment plans.

2.1 PSYCHIATRIC ASSESSMENT

Most elderly patients referred for psychiatric assessment should be seen initially in their own homes. The advantages of this practice include:

1. The patient is seen in the situation with which he or she is familiar.
2. The confusion and disorientation which may be engendered by a trip to hospital, general practice surgery, social services offices or consulting rooms are avoided.
3. The environment can be assessed as well as the patient. Table 2.1 lists some of the important factors in assessment of the home.

Table 2.1 Assessment of the home – some important factors

General level of repair and tidiness of property
Who does the cooking/cleaning/shopping?
Heating, lighting and ventilation
Water supply
Toilet and bathing facilities
Cooking arrangements and food stocks
The stairs
Accident hazards
Sleeping arrangements: has the bed been slept in?
Bottles; other evidence of alcohol abuse
Tablets and medications: as expected or not?

4. The patient's function in his or her own environment and the level of social support can be assessed.
5. Neighbours and relatives are often readily available to give a history of the illness and its impact on them.

Elderly patients who have to be assessed in hospital should be interviewed in a quiet, distraction-free environment, and every effort must be made to put them at ease, otherwise any confusion will be compounded and a falsely pessimistic opinion may be formed.

The patient's family and neighbours often have a key role to play in assessment and continuing management. A good relationship with them is important. At the first interview, the patient and family will have many anxieties, some of which may be founded upon their own ideas about the purpose of the assessment. It is vital to spend time listening to the problems as they are seen by the patient and relatives. A still popular misconception is that the doctor or social worker has come to 'put away' the patient in the local institution. The elderly patient's idea of what institutional care involves may also be quite different from that of the person conducting the assessment. Old people sometimes find it difficult to conceive that an admission to hospital or a residential home could be anything other than permanent. We need to take time to listen to these fears and to explain why we are visiting and the scope and limitations of any help we can offer. Anxiety may inhibit the patient's and relative's ability to grasp and remember what is being said. It may be necessary to repeat the same information several times and to ask questions to clarify whether our explanations have really been understood. Though an assessment may be commonplace to us, for the patient and relative it is often taking place at a crisis point in life. An empathetic manner, acknowledging the patient's and relative's concerns, will help them to realize that their worries have been taken seriously and will help to form a good relationship which is the basis for further treatment.

2.1.1 History

The psychiatric history starts with the presenting complaint (or complaints) including how long it has been present and how it developed. Quite often, the patient lacks insight and believes that nothing is wrong. In these circumstances, careful probing is appropriate. Sometimes, when it is difficult to obtain a clear history of the time course of an illness, things can be clarified by using 'time landmarks' like the previous Christmas or some important personal anniversary. Often, a proper history of the presenting complaint can only be obtained by talking to a friend or relative before or after seeing the patient. In other cases, there may be no relatives available and information may have to be pieced together from a variety of sources such as home-care staff, the social worker and friends and neighbours.

Usually it is best to follow the history of the presenting complaint with an account of the personal history. Old people generally enjoy talking about the past and it is quite easy to introduce the subject. A useful opening line is, 'Tell me a bit about yourself; were you born in these parts?' Memory can be unobtrusively assessed while going through the history by reference to important dates: for example, the date of birth, call-up to the forces and date of marriage. The family history and the history of past physical and nervous complaints can be woven into this brief account of the patient's lifetime and an assessment can be made of their personality and characteristic ways of dealing with stress. Old people, like young people, respond well to those who have a genuine interest in them. Courtesy is vital. It is essential to ensure that the patient can see and hear the interviewer. Talking 'across' patients to other professionals or to relatives generates anxiety and resentment, as does lack of punctuality.

2.1.2 Mental state examination

(a) Level of awareness

At an early stage in the interview, the patient's level of awareness should be assessed. The patient may be drowsy as a result of lack of sleep or medication or because of physical illness. A rapidly fluctuating level of awareness is seen in acute confusional states and a level of awareness that fluctuates from day to day is one of the clues to the diagnosis of chronic subdural haematoma and may also be found in diffuse Lewy-body disease. Impaired awareness can lead to poor function on tests of cognition and memory and, if it is not recognized, can lead to an under-estimation of the patient's true abilities. It is especially important to consider this if the patient is being treated for some recent onset physical problem. The patient's ability to concentrate and pay attention are closely related to level of awareness but may be affected by more mundane things. If the patient is, for example, in pain, it may be very hard for her to understand the relevance of giving an account of her mental state. Disturbance of mood and abnormal perceptual experiences can also impair attention and concentration.

(b) Behaviour

On a home visit the patient's general appearance, behaviour, dress, personal hygiene and the attitude to the interviewer can be observed directly and behaviour can also be deduced indirectly from the state of the house (see Table 2.1). Incontinence can often be smelled and mobility checked by asking the patient to walk a few steps. Especially if the patient lives alone, inconsistencies between appearance and behaviour and the state of cleanliness and organization of the household indicate either that there is a good social support network or that the patient has deteriorated over a relatively short period of time. Various behavioural schedules enable the systematic assessment of the patient's abilities. A shortened form of the Crighton Royal Behavioural Assessment Form is shown in Table 2.2.

It enables a numerical value to be attached to a person's performance in various important areas of behaviour. The advantages of such a scale are that it reminds the assessor of important areas and it enables discrepancies between different

Table 2.2 Modified Crighton Royal Behavioural Scale

Dimension		*Score*
Mobility	Fully ambulant including stairs	0
	Usually independent	1
	Walks with minimal supervision	2
	Walks only with physical assistance	3
	Bed-fast or chair-fast	4
Orientation	Complete	0
	Orientated in ward, identifies persons correctly	1
	Misidentifies persons but can find way about	2
	Cannot find way to bed or toilet without assistance	3
	Completely lost	4
Communication	Always clear, retains information	0
	Can indicate needs, understands simple verbal directions, can deal with simple information	1
	Understands simple information, cannot indicate needs	2
	Cannot understand information, retains some expressive ability	3
	No effective contact	4
Cooperation	Actively cooperative, i.e. initiates helpful activity	0
	Passively co-operative	1
	Requires frequent encouragement or persuasion	2
	Rejects assistance, shows independent but ill-directed activity	3
	Completely resistive or withdrawn	4
Restlessness	None	0
	Intermittent	1
	Persistent by day	2
	Persistent by day, with frequent nocturnal restlessness	3
	Constant	4
Dressing	Correct	0
	Imperfect but adequate	1
	Adequate with minimum of supervision	2
	Inadequate unless continually supervised	3
	Unable to dress or retain clothing	4
Feeding	Correct, unaided at appropriate times	0
	Adequate, with minimum supervision	1
	Inadequate unless continually supervised	2
	Needs to be fed	3

Table 2.2 *Continued*

Continence	Full control	0
	Occasional accidents	1
	Contintent by day only if regularly toileted	2
	Urinary incontinence in spite of regular toileting	3
	Regular or frequent double incontinence	4
Sleep	Normal – no sleeping tablets	0
	Occasional sleeping tablet or occasionally restless	1
	Regular sleeping tablets or restless most nights	2
	Sometimes disturbed despite regular sleeping tablets	3
	Always disturbed at night despite sedation	4

areas of performance to be highlighted so that potentially treatable problems are easily seen and dealt with. It also enables a ready comparison between different patients and between the different points in time for the same patient, even when the assessment is made by a different person. Finally, it gives an overall rating of disability which can be used as a guide to the patient's future needs for care. There are many such scales [1] and they are all imperfect but they do at least enable a quick and systematic approach to the assessment of behaviour. Another useful form is the behavioural assessment form of the Clifton Assessment Procedure for the Elderly [2]. The numerical values ascribed to such scales are, of course, arbitrary. For example, a patient who is disturbed all night may not be manageable at home, despite that factor only contributing four to the total CRBRS score. Scores must therefore be interpreted skilfully taking into account the amount of support available and the peculiar impact of certain behaviours.

(c) Affect (mood)

Mood in the technical sense used by psychiatrists is more than just how we feel. It has been described as 'a complex background state of the organism' and affects not only how we feel but also how we think and even the functioning of our motor and gastrointestinal systems. Old people are not always used to talking about their feelings and it can sometimes be quite difficult to find the right words. Especially where there are communication difficulties, one may have to resort to direct questioning, for example, 'Do you feel happy?' Although patients should always be asked to give an account of their mood, it cannot always be relied upon. Some elderly patients who are quite depressed do not confess to a depressed mood. This may reflect an inability to view the world in psychological terms and is often accompanied by somatization – the presentation of physical (hypochondriacal) complaints. It may also signify a more or less deliberate 'cover up' for fear of hospital admission. 'Anhedonia', loss of the ability to take pleasure in life, is a useful indicator of severe depression. Psychomotor retardation (the slowing of thought and action) can be so profound that patients are unable to report their mood or may even say 'I feel nothing,' though their facial expression, tears, sighs, slowed movement or agitation, may reveal depression. Specific questions should be asked about guilt feelings, money worries, and concerns about health. Where there is depressed mood, careful enquiry should be made about suicidal feelings. This can be introduced in a non-threatening way by a phrase such as, 'Have you ever felt that life was not worth living?' If the patient responds positively to this, further probes can be made about ideas of self-harm. If psychomotor retardation is present, the answer will take some time to come and it is very easy to rush on to the next question before the patient has had time to respond to the previous one. Male sex, depression, living alone, bereavement, long-standing physical illness or disability and alcohol abuse increase the risk.

One group of symptoms is often associated with severe 'biological' depression. This includes early morning wakening, mood worse in the morning and profound appetite loss and weight loss. Self-rating scales such as the Hospital Anxiety and Depression Scale [3] and the Geriatric Depression Scale [4] have been designed to avoid the confusion produced by the use of 'somatic' symptoms in some other scales. However, the frequent somatization of depression in old age may cause 'false negatives' on such scales. The BASDEC [5] is an ingenious card-sort test for rating depression in old age and has been shown to work satisfactorily in elderly medical inpatients.

The opposite of depressed mood is elated mood which is seen in mania and hypomania. In older patients, as in younger patients, decreased sleep, hyperactivity, flight of ideas, thought disorder, irritability and hypersexuality are often prominent symptoms.

Anxiety is common in old age, sometimes in response to the stresses of ageing in our society. Sometimes the patient may be so worried about falling that, in order to avoid anxiety, she restricts her life severely. Thus, a patient who has had one or two falls may, instead of seeking medical help, restrict herself to a downstairs room in the house and never go out. As long as the patient continues to restrict her life, she experiences little anxiety. Whereas in a young person such behaviour would almost certainly lead immediately to the patient being defined as 'sick' and a call for medical attention, in the elderly patient, this restriction is all too easily accepted as 'normal'. When assessing anxiety, attention should therefore be paid not only to how patients feel during the interview (which may, in itself, provoke anxiety!) but also to whether they can engage in the tasks of daily living without experiencing undue anxiety. Anxiety is an affect with physiological accompaniments: a racing pulse, 'palpitations', 'butterflies in the stomach', sweating and diarrhoea. Patients not infrequently use the term 'dizziness' to describe not true vertigo, but a feeling of unreality associated with severe anxiety. Sometimes the physiological changes induced by over-breathing, such as tingling in the arms and even spasm of the muscles of the hand and arm, may make matters worse.

Panic attacks of rapidly mounting anxiety, usually with physiological symptoms, may occur as a part of a phobic disorder, in isolation or, perhaps most commonly in old age, in the context of a depressive disorder.

Phobias occur when the patient is afraid of particular things or situations. Specific phobias (e.g. of spiders or heights) are relatively uncommon and untroublesome in old age but generalized phobias (e.g. fear of going out or of social situations) are relatively common and can be crippling [6].

Perplexity is the feeling which commonly accompanies delirium and may also be found in some mildly demented patients.

The patient with delirium may experience visual or auditory hallucinations and may also be subjected to a whole series of changes in the environment which she cannot properly grasp. The human organism is always trying to make sense of its surroundings and so it is not surprising that patients in this sort of position feel perplexed. It is a useful diagnostic pointer for acute confusional states. The puzzlement ('delusional mood') experienced by some patients early in a schizophrenic illness in some ways resembles the perplexity found in acute confusion, but the other characteristics of acute confusional states (e.g. fluctuating awareness and physical illness) usually make the distinction clear.

(d) Thought (and talk)

The form, speed and content of thought are all assessed. Formal thought disorder occurs in schizophrenia and includes thought-blocking when the patient's thoughts come to an abrupt end, thought withdrawal when thoughts are felt to be withdrawn from the patient's head, and thought insertion. For a fuller description of these phenomena, the reader is referred to a standard textbook of psychiatric phenomenology [7]. Slowing of the stream of thought (thought retardation) is found in many depressive disorders. Slow thinking is also characteristic of some of the organic brain syndromes caused by metabolic deficiencies. Thought is speeded up in mania, often leading to 'flight of ideas' where one thought is built upon another in a way that is founded upon tenuous associations. In dementia, spontaneous thought is often diminished: so-called 'poverty of thought'. The patient with an acute confusional state finds difficulty in maintaining a train of thought because of fluctuating awareness. In dementias of metabolic origin and in some cases of multi-infarct dementia, slowing of thought processes may be accompanied by difficulty in assembling the necessary knowledge to solve particular problems. The observer gets the impression that the patient grasps that there is a problem but is frustrated in trying to cope with it.

Content of thought is influenced by the patient's mood. The depressed patient will often have gloomy thoughts with ideas of poverty or physical illness. The anxious patient's thoughts may be taken up with how to avoid anxiety-provoking situations and there may be unnecessary worries about all aspects of everyday living. The patient who feels persecuted may think of little else. Every noise or happening will be fitted into the persecutory framework. Talk generally reflects the patient's thought, unless suspicion leads to concealment. Speech is also influenced by various motor functions. Slurred speech may be found in the patient who is drowsy or under the influence of drugs or alcohol. Sometimes it also results from specific neurological problems such as a stroke. Patients with multiple sclerosis may produce so-called 'scanning' speech where words are produced without inflexion and with hesitation between words. Patients with severe Parkinsonism may have difficulty in forming sounds at all (aphonia). Some difficulty in finding words and putting speech together is found in many patients with dementia, particularly those with Alzheimer's disease. This is one form of dysphasia. A stream of apparent nonsense, so-called fluent dysphasia, may occur in dementia but is also sometimes associated with a small stroke. The general behaviour of the patient, which is not 'demented', and the sudden onset of the dysphasia, provide important diagnostic clues. Occasionally, fluent dysphasia, especially when it includes new words 'invented' by the patient (neologisms) may be mistaken for the so-called 'word salad' produced by some schizophrenic patients. The sudden onset and absence of other signs of schizophrenia help in diagnosis.

(e) Hallucinations

These can be defined as perceptions without external objects. Visual hallucinations are usually seen in patients with acute confusional states or dementia although occasionally they occur in patients with poor eyesight without measurable organic brain damage, especially if the patient is living alone in a relatively under-stimulating environment. In dementia they are said to be more often found in diffuse Lewy-body disease. Auditory hallucinations (hearing 'voices' or sometimes music or simple sounds) occur in a variety of mental illnesses, especially schizophrenia, where they may consist of a voice repeating the patient's thoughts or of voices talking about the patient in the third person. They also occur in severe depressive illness and mania when they are often in keeping with the patient's mood. Hallucinations of touch (tactile), smell (olfactory) and even taste (gustatory) also occur. Hallucinations of being touched, especially those with sexual connotations, occur in schizophrenia and hallucinations of smell, especially of the patient believing herself to smell 'rotten', in severe depression.

(f) Delusions

A delusion is a false unshakeable belief out of keeping with the patient's cultural background. Delusions occur in fragmentary forms in organic mental states but well-developed delusions are usually found only in schizophrenia and severe affective disorders when ideas of poverty, guilt or illness may develop into absolute convictions. Ideas of persecution are also sometimes found in patients with depression of moderate severity and these, too, can develop into full-blown delusions. Delusions of grandeur, for example that the patient has extraordinary powers of perception or is fabulously rich, are also found in hypomanic states. In paranoid schizophrenia, the delusional content is often very complicated and may involve persecutory activities by whole groups of people. These delusions may be supported by hallucinatory experiences.

(g) Obsessions and compulsions

Obsessions occur when the patient feels compelled to repeat the same thought over and over again. They can be distinguished from schizophrenic phenomena such as thought insertion by the fact that obsessional patients recognize that the thoughts are their own and try to resist them. Sometimes such thoughts may result in compulsive actions, for example, returning many times to check that the door has been locked. Although characteristically a part of obsessive–compulsive disorder, obsessional symptoms also occur in depressed patients and apparently compulsive behaviour can also be a result of memory loss, as when a patient repeatedly checks the door is locked because she has forgotten that she has already done so.

(h) Illusions

Illusions occur when a patient misinterprets a real perception. Some somatic (hypochondriacal) worries can be based on this.

For example, many old people have various aches and pains but sometimes patients may become over-concerned by these and may begin to worry that they indicate some physical illness. Such misinterpretations of internal perceptions are not usually described as illusions although the term would be quite appropriate. Acute confusional states also produce illusions when the patient, seeing the doctor approaching, misinterprets this as someone coming to do him harm and strikes out. This kind of misinterpretation can often be avoided by appropriate management (see Chapters 5 and 9).

(i) Orientation/memory

Orientation for time, place and person should be recorded in a systematic way. The degree of detail would depend upon the time available and the purpose of the examination. Orientation for time can easily be split into gross orientation, for example, the year or approximate time of day (morning, afternoon, evening, night), and finer orientation, for example, the month, the day of the week and the hour of the day. Orientation for person depends upon the familiarity of the person chosen as a point of reference. Orientation for place also depends upon familiarity. A useful brief scale which includes some items of orientation as well as some items of memory-testing is the Abbreviated Mental Test (AMT) score developed by Hodkinson [8] from a longer scale which has been previously correlated with the degree of brain pathology in demented patients. The AMT is reproduced in Table 2.3. A slightly longer related scale

Table 2.3 10-item Abbreviated Mental Test (AMT) score [8]

1. Age
2. Time (to nearest hour)
3. Address for recall at end of test – this should be repeated by the patient to ensure that it has been heard correctly: 42 West Street
4. Year
5. Name of hospital (place seen)
6. Recognition of two people
7. Date of birth
8. Years of First World War
9. Name of present monarch
10. Count backwards 20–1

has been developed for community use [9] though many people 'adapt' the AMT (e.g. by asking the patient's home address rather than hospital name).

Orientation is, to a large extent, dependent upon memory although it should never be forgotten that the patient may not know the name of the hospital she is in, simply because she has never been told. Memory for remote events can be assessed when taking the patient's history. The ability to encode new material can be assessed by the capacity to remember a short address or to remember the interviewer's name. Many patients with dementia will have great difficulty in encoding and storing new memories. Sometimes, especially in the metabolic dementias, one can form the impression that the patient is encoding and storing new material but that they are having great difficulty in retrieving the memory when asked to. This has been described as 'forgetfulness'.

Apraxia, demonstrated in the inability to copy simple drawings and nominal aphasia (the inability to remember the names of common objects) can also be simply tested.

A popular brief assessment of organic mental state is the *Mini-Mental State Examination* [10] which examines memory and a variety of other functions. More detailed descriptions of organic mental state examination can be found in Lishman's *Organic Psychiatry* [11] and Cummings and Benson's *Dementia: a Clinical Approach* [12].

(j) Insight and judgement

In severe psychiatric illness, insight (in the technical psychiatric sense) is often lost. Depressed patients may be unable to accept that they will get better despite remembering many previous episodes of depression which have improved with treatment. Manic and paraphrenic patients may act on their delusions with disastrous consequences. Patients with severe dementia often do not fully realize their plight, which is perhaps fortunate. Patients with milder dementia may have some insight, especially in the metabolic and multi-infarct types of dementia where mood is, not surprisingly, also often depressed. Judgement is related to insight. This can be a particularly difficult question with a moderately demented patient living alone or living with relatives but left alone for a substantial part of the

Table 2.4 Summary of mental state evaluation

Awareness:	level of consciousness, fluctuation; attention and concentration
Behaviour:	general appearance of the patient and her house; behaviour during interview
Affect:	depression (anhedonia), elation, anxiety, perplexity, suicide risk. Somatic changes – sleep pattern, constipation, appetite, weight, in depression. Palpitations, tremor, churning stomach, in anxiety
Thought and talk:	form, speed, content, dysarthria, dysphasia, perseveration
Hallucinations, delusions, obsessions, illusions	
Orientation:	time, place and person
Memory:	remote, ability to encode new information, forgetfulness
Apraxia:	constructional, in daily activities
Nominal dysphasia:	everyday objects in order of increasing difficulty
Judgement and insight	
Other cognitive functions (e.g. arithmetic, proverbs)	
Educational level and intelligence – make due allowance!	

day. Patients may leave gas taps on and be dangerous to themselves and others but at the same time maintain that they are looking after themselves perfectly well and do not need any help, much less residential or nursing-home care. They may have a mistaken image of the care they are refusing. Common sense, professional judgement and interdisciplinary consultation are needed to make decisions in these cases. Consent and legal provisions are discussed further in Chapter 10.

Other tests of cognitive function are considered in the section on neuropsychological assessment. A brief summary of mental state evaluation is given in Table 2.4. It has been put into a mnemonic form for ease of use. The psychiatric history and examination of the elderly patient takes time. It must be tailored to the patient and approached in a sympathetic way. Firing seemingly random questions to test memory and orientation is unlikely to get the best out of the patient. Time taken in proper assessment is not wasted; it avoids treatable illness going untreated or a potentially independent old person being forced into dependency in an institution.

2.1.3 Screening

Screening is used to detect illness at an early stage to enable early intervention. In the UK, GPs are now expected to screen their over-75 year old patients and many are trying simple tests for the two major psychiatric disorders in old age, dementia and depression. The AMT has been used by physicians in geriatric medicine to detect cognitive impairment. It, or similar scales (see above) can be used in the community. For depression, the Geriatric Depression Scale, Hospital Anxiety Depression scale or the BASDEC may be useful, though none has been fully assessed in general practice. Certainly, the low level of detection of depression in old age in general practice needs to be improved, given the exciting prospect of reducing distress and disability opened up by the newer, less toxic anti-depressants and psychological therapies.

2.2 NEUROPSYCHOLOGICAL ASSESSMENT

Neuropsychological assessment is an extension of the kind of brief clinical assessment of memory and other cognitive functions described above. Techniques for neuropsychological assessment are more standardized and time-consuming than the examination described above. They may be justified to assist in difficult diagnoses (though the CAT scan is perhaps more often used these days) or to delineate problems precisely in order to plan a psychological intervention. Similarly, behavioural assessment in psychology is more detailed and specific and more focused on planning interventions than on diagnosis. Because of this the illustrative case histories used in this section include some detail of treatment.The problems that arise from a primary neuropsychological dysfunction are often increased by the personal or interpersonal reaction to the problems and both kinds of assessment are necessary to formulate the patient's problems accurately.

Assessment for cognitive, behavioural, psychodynamic and family therapies is not covered here but is similar to assessment of a young person. Particular issues relevant to psychotherapy with old people are discussed in more detail in Chapter 8.

In elderly people a number of factors alter the interpretation of assessments. These include the effects of ageing on cognitive ability as well as emotional state, vocational opportunities and educational level. One study looked at drawing disability as a measure of constructional apraxia in elderly people with dementia [13] and found that the drawing of a cube, commonly used clinically, was not a useful discriminative test, as many non-demented old people also performed poorly.

Increasingly, general measures of intelligence and personality have been discarded because they do not define specific dysfunction, predict response to treatment or help in planning management. The need to develop normative data for neuropsychological tests with older individuals has been partly mitigated by the production of a number of tests and screening batteries specifically for use with older people. More attention has been paid in recent years to the assessment of dementia and of specific symptoms, such as poor memory. Neuropsychological assessment provides a detailed picture of a person's cognitive strengths and a definition of deficits which is valuable in planning intervention. Although the numbers of trained clinical psychologists working with old people are increasing, in many areas expert neuropsychological assessment may not be available but some of the basic information and methods can be used by other professionals.

2.2.1 Practical issues

Careful selection of candidates for assessment is vital because of the time-consuming and sometimes stressful nature of neuropsychological tests. As with psychiatric assessment, careful preparation, explanation and attention to the setting are essential. Test results can be affected by both internal (emotional) factors including fatigue, anger and anxiety, and external (environmental) factors, such as the expectations and behaviour of others.

The main areas of neuropsychological deficit are outlined in Table 2.5.

Fuller descriptions can be found in standard texts [14, 15].

2.2.2 Standard tests

In the past, standard intelligence tests such as the Weschler Adult Intelligence Scale, were used to test the cognitive func-

Table 2.5 Areas for neuropsychological assessment

Aphasia/dysphasia
This refers to a difficulty in the use of language
Nominal aphasia – the person is able to recognize an object but has difficulty naming it appropriately
Receptive dysphasia – a person may have relatively normal speech but has difficulty in understanding what is being said to her
Expressive – this is an impairment in the production of speech which can range from complete loss to shortened sentences and mild word-finding problems

Agnosia
This refers to an impairment in the ability to recognize things
Visual agnosia – a person is not only unable to name an object but will not be able to recognize it for what it is (unless she uses another sense, e.g. touch)
Spatial agnosia – a person is unable to find her way round familiar surroundings. There may also be distortion in the memory of spatial relationships of her surroundings

Apraxia
This is the impairment of the ability to carry out voluntary and purposeful movements (excluding other causes such as muscle weakness and failure of comprehension)
Constructional apraxia – in this case there is a difficulty in putting together parts to make a whole, e.g. when making a simple drawing
Dressing apraxia – there is a particular difficulty in dressing, e.g. in fastening buttons or tying shoe laces

Frontal
Deficits in this area result in a variety of qualitative signs such as perseveration and emotional lability

Memory
One simple distinction made is between short-term memory (memory for recent events) and long-term memory. An impairment in short-term memory is identified by assessing a person's ability to learn and recall new material over short-time intervals

Acquired knowledge
Difficulties with reading (dyslexia), writing (dysgraphia) and arithmetic (acalculia), which are all acquired abilities, can arise from particular cerebral lesions

Subcortical
This is characterized by forgetfulness, slowness of thought, personality change and the impaired ability to manipulate acquired knowledge

tioning of older adults. The pattern of scores on each scale was compared for adults of different age bands, so that an individual's performance could be compared with that of a group of subjects of similar age. Some psychologists now use a more qualitative and informal approach, which relies on clinical experience, and approximates more to psychiatric assessment.

The observation of the patient's behaviour and language in the initial interview is the starting point. The interviewer takes the history of the patient's problems and listens for difficulties in understanding questions and directions, word finding problems, wandering off the point, repetitiveness and so on. The history also provides information about memory, orientation and cognitive functions such as sequencing. An ordinary magazine can be used as an unthreatening way of testing reading, object and colour recognition, and the use of appropriate words to describe objects [16]. In this way, the stress and inevitable fatigue of the standard 'battery' can be minimized. If the patient is not able or willing to undertake even basic testing, observation can still provide valuable information. One psychologist, faced with a hostile response from a severely disabled and depressed woman, did not attempt formal testing but just talked and listened to her. The woman not only struggled to converse with him, but rewarded him by remembering his name when he saw her again two days later. Observation during ordinary activity, such as dressing or eating, often provides information about spatial abilities, communication skills and apraxia. When specific deficits appear to be present, appropriate formal or informal assessments can be used to delineate them more clearly.

Sometimes specific deficits are put down to 'confusion' or are concealed. A woman was referred who appeared to be inconsistently orientated, with limited but coherent speech. She refused formal interview. Brief observation and interaction showed she was grossly receptively impaired, covering up her impaired understanding of speech with a repertoire of stock phrases and responses to social cues. Previously nobody had considered receptive dysphasia, partly because ordinary assessment procedures did not allow for the possibility and partly because the woman herself tended to conceal the extent of her problems.

The Middlesex Elderly Assessment of Mental State (MEAMS)

[17] is a short test of overall cognitive ability and the Rivermead Behavioural Memory Test [18] assesses memory. Both are designed to assess practical, 'everyday' aspects of function. They produce less exact and comprehensive information than the longer test batteries but this is often outweighed by the ease and speed with which they can be administered, and by their obvious practical relevance.

2.2.3 The environment and assessment

The environment is a major influence on behaviour (Figure 2.1; see also Chapter 5). Where particular neuropsychological deficits exist, based on permanent organic damage, change in behaviour and improvements in the quality of life can still be achieved by offering strategies to compensate for impairments or by changing the environment. Both physical design and modifying interactions with other people can reduce handicap. The analogy of a deaf person can be used: if the physical environment is changed by providing a hearing-aid, and persuading other people to talk more loudly and clearly, the level of handicap can be considerably reduced. Strategies of this sort include instruction on the use of lists, notices, prompts and diaries for managing the effects of memory problems, or information to patient and carers on the effects of the deficit, with help to the carer in judging how and when to offer assistance. Neuropsychological assessment highlights the limitations of some psychiatric diagnoses. Two individuals with the diagnosis of

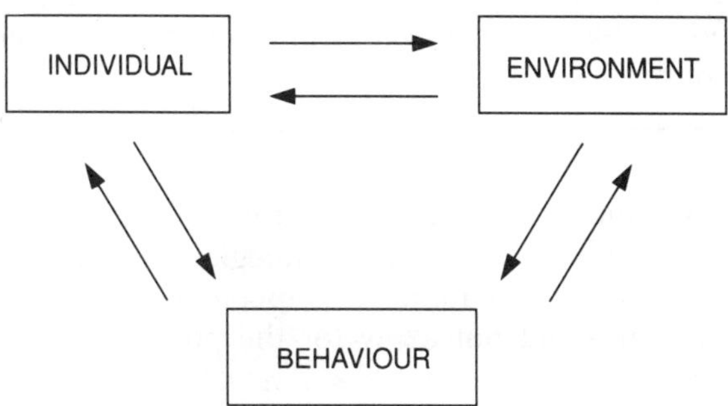

Figure 2.1 The effect of environment on behaviour.

dementia may show different patterns of deficits. One may have a relatively mild impairment of short-term memory, but great difficulty in understanding speech, whereas another may have a severe impairment of short-term memory, but a relatively preserved ability to understand what is being said. In the former patient, the most helpful approach might be to speak in short sentences containing single ideas. In the latter, the patient would probably benefit more from being regularly orientated to time, person and place in a relaxed and non-threatening manner.

Case history 2.1:

Mr G.B. was aged 77 and lived at home with his wife. He was admitted to a medical ward suffering from a suspected occipital stroke. We were consulted about the advisability of discharging him home to his wife after he attacked nursing staff. It turned out that he was both frightened by the stroke and its effects on his perception, and frustrated by his impairment. He returned home on our advice with an agreement to attend day hospital once a week. The management plan shown in Table 2.6 considerably reduced behavioural problems. After several months, he transferred to a Day Centre, and although he initially improved, over the months he showed an intermittent decline, probably indicative of a vascular dementia. He and his wife needed increasing support to manage at home, but in spite of the difficulties they appreciated the flexibility with which help was offered, were confident that they could cope and retained their sense of humour.

This case shows how an understanding of the deficits combined with simple behavioural strategies can help reverse a potentially difficult situation. Attempts to focus on either alone would have been inadequate.

Dysfunction of the frontal lobes may produce a wide range of behavioural consequences, many difficult to identify or quantify. The tearfulness of emotional lability may be miscon-

Table 2.6 Mr G.B.'s management plan

Neuropsychological and behavioural findings	*Management implications*
Right visual field defect	Staff to approach from the left at all times
Poor short-term memory	Routine provision of reality-oriented information and cues (e.g. 'My name is Sheila, it is 12 o'clock and lunch is being served. Can I show you the way?')
Visual agnosia and astereognosis (tactile)	Avoid activities depending on visual and tactile cues and concentrate on other activities such as music
Inappropriate behaviours	Reinforce acceptable behaviour with staff time and interest; reduce reinforcement of inappropriate behaviour
Insight retained (still applies when insight lost)	Treat as an adult; allow choice. Listen and respond to requests. Empathize about loss of abilities
Preserved humour and social skills	Make use of his dry sense of humour

strued as depression, while the presence of disinhibition can lead to a misdiagnosis of hypomania or schizophrenia.

Case history 2.2:

Mrs S.G., a 71-year-old woman, was referred when her husband complained that she was acting out of character. She had begun to swear, seemed more impulsive, and her husband said he found it difficult to reason with her. A psychiatric diagnosis could not easily be made. Frontal signs were found in the absence of global impairment of intellect or other deficits, described in Table 2.7. A CAT scan confirmed the presence of changes in the frontal area. Mr S.G. was offered a session in which he explained the situation at home in detail and was helped to work out strategies for managing the problems identified. When alone, he was able to say just how infuriating and problematic his wife's behaviour had become. She seemed not to be able to think of the effects of her behaviour, nor could she stop herself from doing whatever came into her mind. She perseverated in some actions, and was unable to carry through a series of actions, so that she had become unable to bake or to make a bed. He was advised to offer her prompts at the relevant point in a sequence, and to distract her if she showed signs of restlessness, perseveration or impulsivity. He was also advised on how to do this in a way unlikely to annoy his wife. After trying these measures, he reported that he found it helpful to distract his wife from carrying out some of her impulsive ideas. Distraction also worked when she continued a behaviour inappropriately (perseveration). Giving step-by-step instructions proved more difficult and Mr S.G. discussed more diplomatic ways of offering guidance. These steps improved the quality of the couple's relationship and some of the more hostile behaviours, including the swearing, subsided. Occasional appointments remained necessary to reinforce and modify the strategies and to support the couple.

Table 2.7 Results of Mrs S.G.'s neuropsychological investigation

Neuropsychological findings	*Implications*
Premorbid IQ = present IQ	No intellectual deterioration
Frontal signs:	
Failure on sequencing tasks	
Perseveration	Frontal lobe lesion(s)
Difficulty inhibiting actions	
Difficulty with abstract thought	
Lack of insight	
Emotional lability	

Detailed assessment of neuropsychological functioning and appropriate management measures can produce marked improvements in the behaviour and quality of life of individuals who might otherwise be written off as unhelpable [19].

Case history 2.3:

Mr D.N. was a 66-year-old living at home, supported by relatives who lived next door. He was admitted for assessment following increasing self-neglect. His relatives reported 'slowness rather than silliness'. He had suffered from epilepsy since he was 18 years old. A comparison of the degree and extent of these deficits (Table 2.8) with his score on the Modified Crichton Rating Scale indicated that his behaviour and general functioning were better than might be expected. However, it was still thought that he would not be able to cope with living alone. With his agreement, he was eventually discharged to an old people's home.

Table 2.8 The degree and extent of Mr D.N.'s deficits

Neuropsychological deficit	*Management implications*
Nominal aphasia	Staff to use cueing, e.g. to say first letter or syllable of word he cannot find
Receptive dysphasia	Requests and conversations to include only simple, short sentences with one idea at a time
Subcortical involvement (slowness and occasional irritable outbursts)	Allow him time to complete tasks

One important aspect of Mr D.N.'s management was to make staff aware of his slowness in carrying out tasks, which seemed to be organic in origin, possibly due to subcortical involvement. If this slowness had been interpreted as an inability to carry out or complete the task, the staff might have intervened inappropriately and effectively 'untrained' his self-care skills, making him highly dependent and institutionalized. Because staff at the old people's home were fully informed as to the nature and extent of his deficits, they were able to offer care appropriate to his needs, ensuring that he was given sufficient time to act independently.

2.3 PHYSICAL ASSESSMENT

2.3.1 The importance of working together

Specialists in the psychiatry of old age need to work closely with their medical colleagues, since psychiatric illness in the

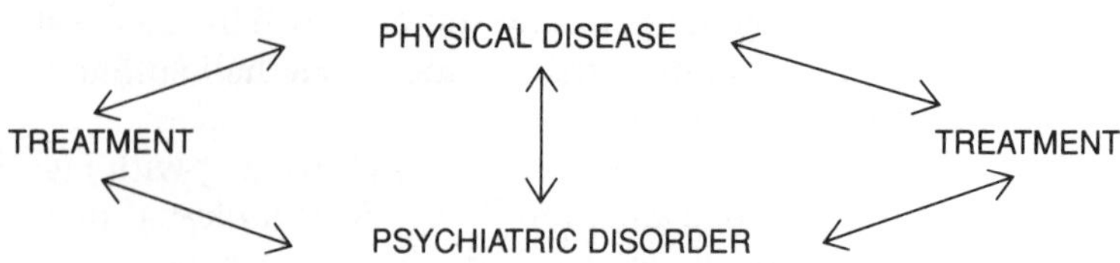

Figure 2.2 Relationships between physical disease and psychiatric disorder.

elderly is often complicated or precipitated by physical illness. Caird and Judge's book [20] on assessment of the elderly patient gives a detailed account of physical assessment to supplement the following brief outline. Figure 2.2 illustrates how treatment for psychiatric disorder can cause physical illness and vice versa. No psychiatric examination, particularly in the elderly, is complete without a physical examination. Even in the patient's home, a selective examination may be carried out though it may be more appropriate to bring the patient to the clinic or the surgery for a more thorough examination. A joint psychiatric–geriatric clinic can facilitate the management of difficult cases.

2.3.2 Sensory impairment

Diminished sensory input, one of the techniques used in 'brain washing', is often inflicted on old people by our slowness in recognizing and correcting defects of sight and hearing. Sensory deprivation may be instrumental in producing paranoid states and in precipitating or worsening confusion. Poor hearing is also associated with depression. Some estimate of visual and auditory acuity is part of the examination of every old person. Wax in the ears is an easily remedied cause of poor hearing. Other forms of deafness may require a hearing-aid. A good deal of patience may be needed to learn to use an aid properly, especially if poor hearing has been present for some time. Look out for flat batteries or dirty battery contacts in hearing-aids. For assessment purposes, more powerful portable amplifiers are useful. Even the inexpensive amplifiers linked to simple headphones advertised in popular magazines can be surprisingly effective. Visual defects vary from those that are easily corrected by spectacles and other aids, to those like cataract and glaucoma that require more complicated surgical or medical intervention.

2.3.3 Medication

Medication for physical and psychiatric disorders is particularly likely to produce side-effects in old people and, unless a careful drug history is taken, these side-effects may be mistaken for a new illness. Anti-hypertensives, digoxin and diuretics may be responsible for depressive symptoms and all drugs with anti-cholinergic effects (including anti-depressants and many anti-psychotics) may produce confusion and constipation among other side-effects. Table 2.9 gives a fuller list of drugs that produce confusion. Benzodiazepines often have a 'hangover' effect and may accumulate over many days to produce confusion. When benzodiazepines are used as hypnotics, they should only be used in short courses. They should not normally be used for anxiety or depression. Postural hypotension induced by tricyclic anti-depressants or anti-psychotics and other drugs may be mistaken for histrionic behaviour and may be dismissed as part of the symptoms of an underlying depressive illness (see Case history 4.4). Many drug interactions occur in old people who are often on a number of different medications. When an elderly patient presents with a new symptom, present medication should always be considered as a possible source of the symptom before further drugs are added.

Table 2.9 Drugs that have been reported to cause or increase confusion in old people

Digoxin	Diuretics
Barbiturates	Non-steroidal anti-inflammatory drugs
Some antibiotics	Benzodiazepines
Tricyclic anti-depressants	Analgesics
Anti-Parkinsonian drugs	Anti-cholinergic drugs
Anti-psychotics	Calcium channel blockers
Anti-histamines	
ACE inhibitors	
Histamine-H2 blockers	

2.3.4 Investigations

Investigations may be planned in the light of findings from the history and examination. There is need for research into the cost-effectiveness of investigations for potentially reversible dementia. Many doctors would confine themselves to haemoglobin, full blood count and film, urea and electrolytes and thyroid function tests; some would routinely add serum B12 and folate and a serological test for syphilis, though the necessity for the last is disputed. Other tests such as chest X-ray, skull X-ray, Electroencephalogram, radio-isotope brain scan computerized axial tomography (CAT) and other forms of brain scan are at present only justified by specific indications. Hopes that CAT might provide an easy and definitive diagnosis of senile dementia by demonstrating brain atrophy have not been realized due to wide overlaps in the picture between normal, functionally ill and demented patients, though occasionally a scan will turn up an unsuspected tumour or other problem. Newer scanning techniques such as Nuclear Magnetic Resonance [21] or Positron Emission Tomography may eventually be able to help in definitive diagnosis before death but the research potential has yet to be realized in routine clinical practice.

2.4 SOCIAL ASSESSMENT

2.4.1 Quantitative assessment

The quality and quantity of relationships need to be considered. The quantity of relationships can easily be summarized in a social network diagram [22]. In our adaptation of this (Figure 2.3a,b), a box is drawn which contains the name of the patient and members of their household, together with a brief note of the type of accommodation. Down one side of the box the timing of visits by friends and family who live outside the household are noted, and down the other, the timing of services such as home care, warden, meals-on-wheels service, etc. The base of the box is used for visits out of the household by the patient. Case history 2.4 illustrates how the social network diagram can be used not only to summarize current arrangements but to plan their improvement.

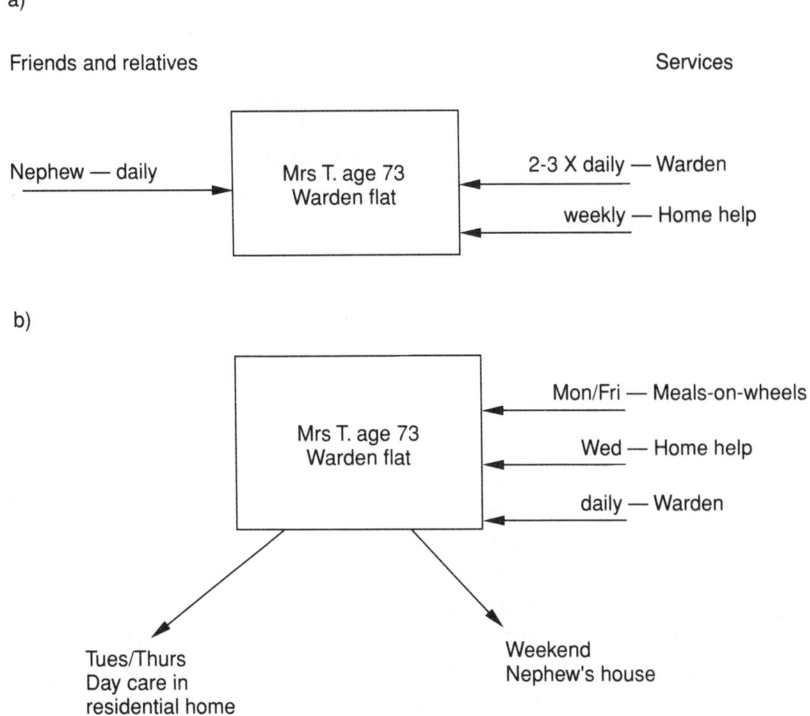

Figure 2.3 The social network diagram a) before intervention b) after intervention.

Case history 2.4:

This 73-year old widow, living alone, presented to the physicians in geriatric medicine with repeated falls. Investigations showed no cause for the falls and she was managed symptomatically. About 18 months after the initial assessment it became evident that she was abusing alcohol and that this was the cause of her falls. The nephew discovered a cache of empty brandy bottles under the sink with a number of different brand names that were unwittingly supplied by a number of helpers, each of whom thought he or she was the patient's only source of supply! Psychiatric assessment revealed she had started to abuse alcohol for the first time in late life in a misguided attempt to relieve depression following the loss of her husband. After a period of inpatient withdrawal and treatment for nutritional deficiency and depression, her social network was reorganized in a way that helped her successfully to fill her life with activities other than drinking alcohol (see Figure 2.3b).

2.4.2 Qualitative assessment

The quality of relationships can be assessed indirectly from the past history of the patient and family and more directly during a joint interview. It is worth trying to assess what each member of the family is aiming for and how open family members are in their communication with each other. Sometimes there is a pathological attachment between family members resulting in a maladaptive pattern of caregiving. The growing dependence, physical and psychological of old people with progressive illnesses such as Parkinson's disease and Alzheimer's dementia can put extraordinary stress on family relationships that will reveal previously carefully disguised 'fault lines'. Skill in family therapy can best be developed in supervised practice and there are now a few units in the UK taking an interest in this work. Traps for inexperienced workers include collusion in the pattern of family relationships or ill-timed, unproductive confrontation. Because services are sometimes only made available when a crisis has occurred and the family are at the end of their tether, we do see relatives who may be labelled as 'rejecting'. This happens less frequently than it used to since the development of more effective services leads to earlier intervention before a crisis has occurred. Even when a crisis has occurred, it may be possible to manage it in such a way that the relatives realize that they can continue to cope with the help of appropriate services.

2.4.3 Making allies of the family

An important factor here is a prompt response, usually in the form of a home visit. This is the first step in impressing the family that help is available. Carers are relieved to find someone who has time and is willing to listen to the problems they are facing and provide practical help. This can cause family members to re-evaluate their attitudes and avoid premature decisions to put an elderly relative into care. The understanding and assessment that family members make of a situation may be quite different from the professional viewpoint and must be 'heard' and respected by the team that is planning help. The appropriate use of short-term hospital admission, day care, family care and home-care services to relieve perceived strains can enable the family to cope. Work with the family is considered further in Chapter 8.

2.4.4 The need for 24-hour care

When an old person lives alone and suffers from moderate or severe dementia, it may be impossible to provide adequate supervision without admission to a long-stay care facility. This should not be viewed as a 'failure' to keep the person 'in the community' but as the appropriate use of one of a range of options for providing care. Management depends upon psychiatric and medical diagnosis as well as the family and social situation and it is in understanding the various components of the situation and how they interact in order to produce the best possible management plan that the skill of the psychogeriatric team resides.

2.5 THE BALANCING ACT

The old person living at home can be considered to be performing a delicate balancing act (Figure 2.4). The old person in this illustration balances on a three legged stool. The legs are her physical, psychological and social 'health'. If any of the legs are taken away, the person falls into ill health, in a manner which may not appear directly related to the underlying cause. Case history 2.4 illustrated this well. The underlying problem was unresolved grief and loneliness, leading to depression and excessive drinking; but the initial presentation was to the medical services with falls. Case history 2.5 provides a further illustration.

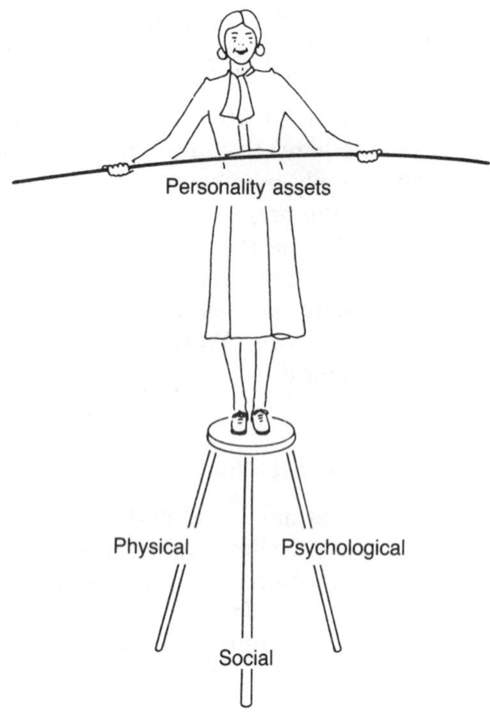

Figure 2.4 The balancing act.

Case history 2.5:

An elderly widow, living alone, suddenly became breathless. Her family doctor thought that she might have had a mild heart attack a few days previously and decided to manage her at home. Two days later, she became acutely disturbed, barricading herself in her room and hurling abuse (and small items of furniture) at those who tried to help her. The family doctor made a correct diagnosis of acute confusional state secondary to her physical illness. She was unable to secure a medical admission because of the patient's confusion but managed to admit her to a psychiatric unit for old people where medical treatment of her heart failure produced a rapid improvement in her mental state.

Hopefully, closer co-operation between medical and psychiatric services for old people means this patient would be accepted for medical admission today.

2.6 PROBLEM FORMULATION AND MANAGEMENT

Each patient needs a 'tailor-made' plan of medical, psychological and social management. This will often need to be agreed on a multi-disciplinary basis after assessments by several different members of the team. Many teams insist that the initial assessment is by a senior member of medical staff since physical and psychiatric illness usually need to take precedence in any management plan. Another member of the team may attend with the doctor or later. In any case, it is essential that the initial assessment includes an overall view of medical, psychological and social factors and that the family are given some idea of the likely management and the available help at that first assessment. This includes at least an outline knowledge of local home care, day care, voluntary groups, financial allowances and other relevant sources of help. The care plan will usually evolve and develop as the patient's condition and circumstances change. The care-planning procedures [23] that local authorities in the UK have been asked to agree with health authorities formalize this process. They introduce a more carefully monitored procedure to replace the informal approach that has prevailed until now. There are dangers of bureaucratic inflexibility and slowness replacing the more rapid and flexible team approach. Case management is a related philosophy which social services departments introduced in April 1993. This approach potentially allows a more flexible deployment of resources, though there is a danger that it will simply become a crude bureaucratic mechanism to control costs and transfer blame.

2.6.1 Timing and teamwork

A medical and psychosocial 'diagnosis' is only the beginning of patient management. Because of the multiplicity of problems faced by patients, a haphazard approach to management is time-wasting, inefficient and potentially dangerous. For example, arranging long-term home care support for people who are suffering from undiagnosed and untreated depressive episodes

CARE PROGRAMME INFORMATION FORM:
DATE OF MEETING/REVIEW [01 | 08 | 93] MEETING/REVIEW NO. [1]
PREVIOUS MEETING/REVIEW NO. [ ]

PATIENT DATA:

NAME & INITS: Smith J
GENDER: (MALE) FEM
D.O.B: ______
SECTION 117 APPLIES: YES/NO

ADDRESS: 3 Brook Close
Anytown
PATIENT ORIGIN: IN/PT : DAY PT : (COMMUNITY) :
(please ring)
ETHNIC ORIGIN (British) : European : Afro-Carribean : Black African
(please ring) Indian Sub Continent : Other :

POST CODE: AN3 6BJ

PATIENT CONSENTS TO CARE PROGRAMME : (YES) NO

DATE CARE PROGRAMME COMMENCED [01 / 08 / 93]

DATE CARE PROGRAMME COMPLETED [: :]

CARE PROGRAMME DATA:

NO.	PATIENT'S NEEDS AND	INTERVENTIONS:
1	Depressed mood	Antidepressant
2	Recurrent depression	Lithium (OPD to check)
3	Bereavement	Counselling from CPN
4	Sheltered housing	Soc. Services to
5		support application
6		Home Care (pro temps)
7		

NO.	OUTCOME OF INTERVENTIONS (indicate if need was met or unmet)	MET/UNMET
1		
2		
3		
4		
5		
6		
7		

SOURCES OF SUPPORT:

AFTER CARE COORDINATOR: Name & Designation: Anne Barton (CPN)
Contact Tel. No: 0946 00000

SOCIAL SERVICES WORKER: Name & Designation: Mike Busby
Contact Tel. No: 0946 00001

HEALTH SERVICES KEY WORKER: Name & Designation: Community Nurse (as above)
Contact Tel. No: ______

CONSULTANT: J. Watt GP: F. Rodney

PRIMARY INFORMAL CARER: Pat Bloggs (daughter)

OTHER INVOLVEMENTS: Home Care

DATE OF NEXT REVIEW: ___ / ___ / ___

Figure 2.5 The care-planning form.

may 'keep them going' in the community but does not permit them to lead the best possible quality of life, and may lead to a treatment-resistant depressive illness or even to suicide. Arranging nursing home care for people whose confusion is due to an undiagnosed medical condition denies them proper treatment, reduces their independence, wastes resources and may also have fatal consequences. On the other hand, a narrowly medical approach to people's problems will also reduce their prospects of independent living. If the patient in Case history 2.4 had not been managed with attention to the social and emotional factors underlying the alcohol abuse, it is much more likely that the abuse would have recurred, producing permanent physical or mental damage.

Teamwork is therefore essential and it is most important that case management and care-planning procedures do not detract from the tradition of multi-disciplinary teamwork that has been built up in many psychogeriatric services.

The traditional psychiatric formulation of a patient's problems has always included not only the psychiatric diagnosis but also all relevant medical, psychological and social factors. Care plans do the same by listing the patient's needs, planning interventions to meet those needs and agreeing responsibility between professionals and agencies for different components of the plan. Figure 2.5 gives an example of a care-planning form with the sort of needs and interventions that might be agreed. Though these plans are ideally agreed at a meeting of patient, caregiver(s), health service and social services staff, in practice we have found this too time-consuming to be accommodated within available resources. Now we reserve full meetings for difficult cases and use an abbreviated (though still firmly multi-disciplinary) procedure for the majority of cases. Community team members review patients regularly but only reformulate plans and involve other disciplines in this as and when circumstances demand.

2.7 CONCLUSION

This chapter has dealt with the various aspects of assessment in psychiatric disorder in old people and how these can be brought together to formulate an overall care plan for the patient. It has advocated a flexible team approach rather than a bureaucratic procedural approach to this challenging task. This is based on the fundamental premise that multi-disciplinary teams can work effectively and that individuals within those teams work best when management sets them free to do the work they have been trained to do. Teams should not be constrained by over-detailed and time-consuming procedures that will inevitably result in a reduction in the quality and/or the quantity of service that can be provided within existing resources.

REFERENCES

1. Israel, L., Kozarevic, B. and Sartorius, N. (1984) *A Source Book of Geriatric Assessment*, WHO/S, Karger, Basle.
2. Pattie, A. and Gilleard, C. (1979) *Manual of the Clifton Assessment Procedure for the Elderly* (CAPE), Hodder & Stoughton Educational, Sevenoaks.
3. Kenn, C., Wood, H., Kucyj, M. *et al.* (1987) Validation of the Hospital Anxiety and Depression Rating Scale (HADS) in an elderly psychiatric population. *International Journal of Geriatric Psychiatry*, **2**, 189–93.
4. Yesavage, J., Brink, T., Rose, T. *et al.* (1983) Development and validation of a geriatric depression screening scale: a preliminary report. *Journal of Psychiatric Research*, **17**, 37–49.
5. Adshead, F., Day Cody, D. and Pitt, B. (1992) BASDEC: a novel screening instrument for depression in elderly medical inpatients. *British Medical Journal*, **305**, 397.
6. Lindesay, J. (1991) Phobic disorders in the elderly. *British Journal of Psychiatry*, **159**, 531–41.
7. Sims, A.C. (1988) *Symptoms in the mind: an introduction to descriptive psychopathology*. Baillière, London.
8. Hodkinson, H.M. (1972) Evaluation of a mental test score for assessment of mental impairment in the elderly. *Age and Ageing*, **1**, 233–8.
9. Kay, D.W., Black, S.E., Blessed, G. *et al.* (1992) The prevalence of dementia in a general practice sample: upward revision of reported rate after follow-up and reassessment. *International Journal of Geriatric Psychiatry*, **5**, 179–86.
10. Folstein, M.F., Folstein, S.E. and McHugh, P.R. (1975) 'Mini-Mental State'. A practical method for grading the cognitive state of patients for the clinician. *Journal of Psychiatric Research*, **12**, 189–98.
11. Lishman, W.A. (1987) *Organic Psychiatry: the Psychological Consequences of Cerebral Disorder*, Blackwell Scientific Publications, Oxford.
12. Cummings, J.L. and Benson, D.F. (1983) *Dementia, a Clinical Approach*, Butterworth, Boston.

13. Moore, V. and Wyke, M.A. (1984) Drawing disability in patients with senile dementia. *Psychological Medicine*, **14**, 97–105.
14. Hart, S. and Semple, J.P. (1990) *Neuropsychology and the Dementias*. Taylor and Francis, London.
15. Walsh, R.W. (1978) *Neuropsychology: a Clinical Approach*. Churchill Livingstone, Edinburgh.
16. Holden, U.P. and Woods, R.T. (1988) *Reality Orientation: Psychological Approaches to the 'Confused' Elderly*, Churchill Livingstone, Edinburgh.
17. Golding, E. (1989) *The Middlesex Elderly Assessment of Mental State*, Thames Valley Test Company, Bury St Edmunds.
18. Wilson, B., Cockburn, J. and Baddeley, A. (1985) *The Rivermead Behavioural Memory Test*, Thames Valley Test Company, Bury St Edmunds.
19. Hanks, H. and Martin, C. (1988) Psychological assessment and treatment, in *Rehabilitation of the 'Physically Disabled Adult*, (ed. C.J. Goodwill and M.A. Chamberlain), Croom Helm, London.
20. Caird, F.I. and Judge, T.G. (1979) *Assessment of the Elderly Patient*, Pitman Medical Publishing, Tunbridge Wells.
21. Brown, G.G., Levine, S.R., Gorell, J.M. *et al.* (1989) In vivo 31 P NMR profiles of Alzheimer's disease and multiple subcortical infarct dementia. *Neurology*, **39**, 1423–7.
22. Capildeo, R., Court, C. and Rose, F.C. (1976) Social network diagram. *British Medical Journal*, **i**, 143–4.
23. Department of Health (1990) Joint Health/Social Services Circular: Health and Social Services (Development: *'Caring for People', the Care Programme Approach for People with a Mental Illness Referred to the Specialist Psychiatric Services*, HC(90)23/LASSL(90)11, Department of Health Publications Unit, London.

3

The classification of mental illness in old age

This book adopts a problem-solving approach rather than one based solely on diagnosis. The chapters on the presentations of mental illness in old age are arranged with this in mind. Nevertheless, the diagnosis and classification of mental illness are very important if we are to recognize diseases that may respond to specific treatments and in order to test out new methods of treatment. One of the criticisms of much early evaluation of drugs in dementia was that the dementia itself was not identified according to its probable causes. More recent research has attempted to distinguish clinical Alzheimer's disease from vascular dementia. There are some doubts as to how reliably this can be done and in addition, the new diagnostic entity of diffuse Lewy-body dementia (see later) is now further confusing the picture.

All disciplines working with old people need to look beyond the presenting problem to its underlying cause or causes. In medicine this involves paying attention to the symptoms the patient presents with and to the history of their evolution in an attempt to reach a diagnosis – a medical explanation of the underlying causes of the problem. Doctors who respond to the patient's symptoms without attention to diagnosis may harm patients, by allowing underlying illness to progress untreated. One of the authors had the misfortune, some years ago, to come across a severely depressed man whose general practitioner had labelled him as 'confused' and who had been prescribed two different laxatives and an anti-diarrhoeal drug. In fact, he was depressed and the depression had led to severe constipation with secondary incontinence. He responded to treatment based on appropriate psychiatric and physical diagnosis.

There is a risk that the classification of disease, pursued as an end in itself, can lead to the human needs of the patient being ignored. On the other hand, the failure to analyse and classify can lead to inappropriate, unhelpful and even harmful treatment.

3.1 CLASSIFICATION

The idea that all mental illness in old age is due to senile degeneration remains popular. It is only since the Second World War that the classification of mental disorder in old age has begun to be understood. In 1956 Roth [1], in a classic research report, described how elderly psychiatric inpatients with different diagnoses had different prognoses measured in simple outcome terms at six months and two years. The measures of outcome he used were crude: whether the patient was dead, living in an institution or back at home. The diagnostic categories he looked at in his hospital-based study were: senile psychosis, more recently often referred to as senile dementia (Alzheimer's type or late-onset dementia in Alzheimer's disease), arteriosclerotic psychosis (vascular dementia), delirium (acute confusional states), paraphrenic illnesses and depressive illness. Roth's approach to diagnosis was descriptive. He looked for factors in the mental state and previous history which pointed to a diagnosis and then confirmed the validity of the diagnosis by looking at the natural history of the illness. Medical diagnosis is generally based on such a descriptive approach, but additional help is given in classification by the response to different treatments of different disease categories. Ultimately, pathological, biochemical or psycho-social causation, where one or more of these can be established, sets the seal on diagnostic classification.

Since the first edition of this book there have been advances in the classification used for mental illnesses. The *International Classification of Diseases* tenth edition (ICD10) [2] is more useful on old age than were previous editions, though there are still some areas where the unique presentations of disease in old age are not adequately taken into account. The American Psychiatric Association's Diagnostic and Statistical Manual (fourth edition – DSMIV), due to be published soon, will probably follow ICD10 closely. The broad divisions of ICD10 will be used in this text and ICD10 classifications for the terms we use will be given to enable the interested reader to look up details in the ICD10 glossary. Brief descriptions of the main diagnostic categories follow. Expanded descriptions have been given for conditions not covered in later chapters.

3.1.1 Organic mental disorders (ICD10; F00–F09)

These conditions are usually believed to be based on structural changes in the brain. They affect around ten per cent of people over the age of 65 years.

(a) Dementia in Alzheimer's disease – late onset (AD, ICD10; F00.1)

This accounts for around half of psychiatric hospital inpatients dying with dementia and probably (if the complication introduced by diffuse Lewy-body dementia is ignored) a similar proportion of those in the community. It is a condition of insidious onset usually presenting with memory loss and progressing slowly to personality deterioration and the impairment of self-care abilities. The anatomical and biochemical pathology are increasingly understood but the underlying causes have not been identified, although they almost certainly involve the interaction of genetic susceptibility and environmental factors. Technically, AD is a diagnosis based on microscopic examination of the brain after death and some people prefer the term *probable* Alzheimer's disease for the clinical syndrome.

(b) Vascular dementia (ICD10; F01)

Vascular dementia affects around 20 per cent of elderly people with dementia. It can be divided into three main sub-types: **vascular dementia of acute onset** (F01.0) which develops rapidly after a series of strokes or a single large infarct; **multi-infarct dementia** (MID; F01.1), more gradual in onset, following a number of small strokes; and **subcortical vascular dementia** (F01.2) where the clinical picture more closely resembles AD. About a further fifth of dementias are due to a mixture of AD and vascular disease. Recently it has been suggested that up to a third of cases diagnosed clinically and even neuropathologically as AD have pathology related to that found in Parkinson's disease with diffuse Lewy bodies. There is dispute as to whether this is a distinct subgroup of AD or merely a coincidental finding [3, 4].

(c) Other dementias

This group includes other dementias with an hereditary component such as Pick's disease, dementias associated with space-occupying lesions and dementias with metabolic causes, B12 deficiency, thyroid deficiency, etc., which overlap with some of the causes of delirium (acute confusional states). The dementias and delirium are discussed in more detail in Chapter 5.

3.1.2 Schizophrenia and related disorders (ICD10; F20–29)

These affect only about one per cent of old people. Many people with schizophrenia of early onset survive into old age. Until recently, the needs of these people have been hidden in our large mental institutions. As newer generations of schizophrenic patients are cared for in the community, they often need special help when the problems of old age are added to their underlying illness. Late-onset schizophrenia nearly always takes the form of a paranoid illness and is discussed in Chapter 7.

3.1.3 Mood (affective) disorders (ICD10; F30–39)

The severe forms of affective illness have a partly genetic and biochemical aetiology although the later the first onset of disease, the less important are the genetic factors. They have been divided into **manic episodes** (F30), **bipolar affective disorder** (F31), **depressive episodes** (F32), **recurrent depressive disorder** (F33), and **persistent mood disorder**.

Manic episodes in old age nearly always occur in the context of recurrent episodes of affective disorder. Sometimes after many years of recurrent depression, the first episode of mania occurs in old age [5]. A possible reason for this is an increased incidence of (non-dementing) brain damage. These illnesses are discussed more fully in Chapter 4. **Persistent mood disorder** includes **dysthymia** (F34.1), roughly equivalent to the older concept of depressive neurosis.

3.1.4 Neurotic, stress-related and somatoform disorders (ICD10; F40–48)

It is not certain how common these disorders are in late life. **Phobic anxiety disorders** (F40) in old age have been closely studied recently [6]. Phobias are found in six to ten per cent of old people but rarely present to doctors. Old people with phobic disorders report higher rates of specific and non-specific neurotic symptoms and more previous chronic psychiatric disorder compared to mentally well old people. They have higher rates of contact with general practitioners and need more help in personal care from their families. Most have more than one fear. About half of all phobias in old age are of the **agoraphobic** (F40.0) type and these are by far the most disabling. People with agoraphobia are abnormally frightened to leave home, to enter shops or crowded places or to travel alone. In old age, this condition is predominantly of late onset and attributed to an episode of physical illness or other traumatic event. It causes moderate or severe social impairment whereas **specific phobias** (F40.2) – e.g. the fear of spiders – are associated with earlier onset and minimal social impairment. Old people with **agoraphobia** are more likely to have lost a parent in childhood and may have associated depressive symptoms. Other conditions such as **panic disorder** (F41.0), **generalized anxiety disorder** (F41.1), **obsessive compulsive disorder** (F42), **adjustment reactions** (F43), **dissociative** – formerly called **hysterical or histrionic** – **disorders** (F44) and **somatoform** disorders (F45 – see Chapter 6) all exist in old age but are less often recognized than they should be. Roughly speaking, about half of people with these disorders have had symptoms all their adult lives but another half develop their symptoms for the first time in response to the stresses of late life. Caution must be exercised in diagnosing these conditions, since many of the symptoms associated with them are also found in mood disorders. If in doubt it is always worth considering a psychiatric assessment, since depressive episodes are relatively easy to treat with modern anti-depressants and since some of the other disorders above (e.g. panic disorder and obsessive compulsive disorder) sometimes also respond well to anti-depressant treatment.

3.1.5 Personality disorder (F60)

This term is often used in a perjorative way. Personality is hard to define. It describes an habitual style of behaviour but there is debate over how constant personality is and how far it is influenced by situational factors. Theories about the maturation of personality after early adulthood are not well developed, though Erikson (see Chapter 1) has described the core maturational task of late life as being that of establishing ego-integrity or facing despair. Many different personality traits and types have been described by various authors, and interest in their relevance to mental disorder has been revived by the use of multi-axial diagnosis in recent editions of the American Psychiatric Association's *Diagnostic and Statistical Manuals* (DSMIII and DSMIIIR).

The most useful short definition of personality disorder from a clinical point of view is that of a long-standing pattern of maladaptive interpersonal behaviour. Behaviour is an important marker because it can be observed. As people age, changes in physical status and health militate against various kinds of behaviour often associated with personality disorder in younger people. Impulsive behaviour, law-breaking, initiating fights, promiscuity and aggression to children are all less likely for a variety of reasons. While some behaviour which acts as a marker of disorder in younger people is less likely to be found in older people, other 'marker' behaviour such as social withdrawal may become more likely because of physical or sensory disabilities or undiagnosed illness, including depressive illness.

Social expectations of behaviour also change. An old man who strikes another person is probably less likely to be charged with assault than a young man who does the same. An old woman who behaves histrionically is less likely to be labelled 'hysterical' than a young woman. We all have socially conditioned expectations about what is 'normal' for people in different age groups and of different gender which influence where we draw the line between 'normal' and 'abnormal'.

Early studies found a prevalence of about four per cent for 'character disorders', including paranoid states [7], in old age, though how far this accords with modern concepts of personality disorder is not clear. Doctors' diagnostic habits may be responsible for apparent differences in prevalence between younger and older people. One recent study of psychiatric inpatients found seven per cent of old people were given an additional diagnosis of personality disorder compared with 30 per cent of younger patients. Traits, not amounting to 'disorder' were found in 16 per cent of the elderly and four per cent of the younger group. Four-fifths of the diagnoses in elderly people were accounted for by **dependent** (F60.7), **histrionic** (F60.4) and **compulsive** (**anankastic** F60.5: ICD10) personality with dependent personality alone accounting for over half. In the younger group, the personality diagnoses were distributed more widely between the different personality diagnoses. Personality problems are more common in those with depressive illness in old age and avoidant, dependent and compulsive traits are particularly likely to occur in these patients, irrespective of age, with some increase in compulsive traits in old age. **Dissocial** (**antisocial**) **personality disorder** (F60.2) occurs in older people but is often contained within the family, sometimes only emerging when the person has to go into residential care which is not as tolerant of antisocial behaviour as some families!

Personality and behaviour disorders due to brain disease (F07) occur in dementia and may include some antisocial characteristics. In Alzheimer's disease changes are often found and correspond to four different patterns: 1) initial change followed by a period of stability; 2) continuing change throughout the course of the illness; 3) no major change, and 4) emergence of disturbed behaviour which then regresses as the dementia develops [8]. Patients with Alzheimer's and vascular dementia were rated by their spouses as more out of touch, reliant on others, childish, listless, changeable, unreasonable, lifeless, unhappy, cold, cruel, irritable and mean than mentally well spouses. Some of these perceived changes may be due to the spouse's reaction to the illness, some might be directly determined by organic change and others might mark a reaction of the person to the experience of dementia.

Personality problems are often the result of disturbed relationships in earlier life. Despite such damage, people will often cope well with life provided they are not exposed to abnormal stress. Case history 3.1 illustrates these points.

Some personality patterns can be identified that fall short of frank personality disorder. Insecure, rigid and anxiety-prone

Case history 3.1:

Mrs M.S. was a 68-year-old widow. At the age of four her mother died, allegedly as a result of a beating from her husband (although he was never prosecuted). A cause of this beating was that Mrs M.S. was an illegitimate child of her mother's lover, conceived while her father was away during the First World War. After her mother's death Mrs M.S. was turned out on the street, and taken in by another family. She says they used to go out drinking a lot. At the age of 17 she went into hospital with TB and subsequently married a man who flew into unexpected rages, and was later diagnosed as having schizophrenia. She looked after him for many years, but in 1976 he finally went into a hostel. She blamed herself for not looking after him adequately, perhaps reflecting her own feelings of having received inadequate care in childhood, and had a 'breakdown'. After that, she lived a nomadic life staying in boarding houses at various seaside resorts, never very satisfied with her lot, and always anxious and frightened. When seen in 1985, she had returned to her home town, and was about to be ejected from the boarding house in which she was living. She had some mild biological signs of depression and unrealistic expectations that the social services could immediately find her permanent accommodation near her sister. After a further journey to another seaside town, she was admitted for treatment of her depression and assessment of what help could be given for her maladaptive responses to stress. The diagnostic label of **anxious (avoidant) personality disorder** (F60.6) could be attached to this lady but although technically correct, it does little justice to the way she coped for years with a schizophrenic husband. After a period of six months in hospital during which staff refused to confirm her 'life-script' by rejecting her, despite awkwardness on her part about finding new accommodation, she was rehoused and followed up in the community by a member of our team, perhaps at last finding the consistent caregiving she had been missing most of her life.

people have the greatest problems in adapting to old age and seem especially prone to develop depressive symptoms. Paranoid, isolated people have a greater risk of developing paranoid illnesses but often cope well unless physical or psychiatric symptoms require outside help. Such people will often refuse help and may end up living in squalid and unhealthy circumstances. Passively dependent people cope well as long as they have someone to depend on, but they are vulnerable to the loss of a spouse or other caring person. See Kroessler [9] for a full review of personality disorder in old age.

3.1.6 Alcoholism and drug-related disorders (F10–F19)

These are largely hidden problems in old age. We still occasionally come across old people who are dependent on barbiturates prescribed for the first time as sleeping tablets many years ago, though dependence on sleeping tablets of the benzodiazepine group (see Chapter 9) is now more of a problem. Those atypical elderly depressed patients who respond dramatically to non-selective mono-amine oxidase inhibitors may need to continue them indefinitely. In this case a kind of 'dependence' may be a reasonable price to pay for a great improvement in the quality of life. Conventional tricyclic antidepressants and the newer anti-depressant compounds do not seem to produce dependence syndromes but there is still a risk of relapse of the depression when they are stopped. As will be apparent from the above, drug dependence in old people is usually related to prescribed drugs and both its causes and cure are in the hands of doctors.

The belief persists that alcohol abuse and dependence are rarely, if ever, seen in old age. The present generation of old people drink less alcohol than their younger contemporaries, but this may be misleading for several reasons. First, owing to differences in average body composition, old people may need less alcohol to become intoxicated [10]. They may also respond differently to survey methods and present figures do not rule out the possibility of a cohort effect as our current generation of heavy drinkers grows older. An epidemiological study in London [11] has shown that for women the prevalence rate for alcoholism continues to rise into the seventh decade whereas for men it peaks in the fifties. Two groups of elderly alcoholics are discernible: those chronic alcoholics who have survived into late life and those, often women, who have turned to alcohol for the first time in response to the stresses of ageing (see Case history 2.4). Often old people with alcohol problems present with falls, self-neglect or unexplained confusion. Sometimes they develop a withdrawal delirium after hospital admission precipitated by some other problem. Their alcohol intake may be concealed by themselves and unknown to, or concealed by, family and friends. Mobility problems may cause them to rely on others for supply. These others may be innocent friends or relatives who are an unwitting part of a large supply network as in Case history 2.4 or they may be other alcoholics. If these other alcoholics are close friends or family members, then the prognosis for the old person's alcoholism is worsened. If an old person is admitted to hospital and friends or family members come in drunk, then the possibility that the old person, too, has alcohol problems should be explored. Old people with such problems are especially vulnerable to economic exploitation by other alcoholics, partly because of their frequent dependence on such people for supply of the alcohol and partly because increasing age is a major risk factor for the development of alcoholic dementia with impaired judgement and disinhibition. Late-onset elderly alcoholics with clear social precipitants respond relatively well to help provided they are willing to accept social change. Chronic alcoholics, especially if they live in an alcoholic culture, are especially difficult to help. A fuller discussion of alcohol abuse in old people is found in *Reviews in Clinical Gerontology* [12].

3.2 CONCLUSION

This chapter has dealt with the classification of mental disease in old age using the ICD10 system of classification adopted by the World Health Organization. The following chapters will deal with some of the main presentations of psychiatric disorder in old people and the last few chapters will discuss psychological and medical treatment in its legal and cultural setting.

REFERENCES

1. Roth, M. (1956) The natural history of mental disorder in old age. *Journal of Mental Science*, **101**, 281–301.
2. World Health Organization (1992) *The ICD-10 Classification of Mental and Behavioural Disorders: Clinical Descriptions and Diagnostic Guidelines*, World Health Organization, Geneva.
3. Byrne, E.J. (1992) Diffuse Lewy-body disease: disease, spectrum disorder of variety of Alzheimer's disease? *International Journal of Geriatric Psychiatry*, **7**, 229–34.
4. Birkett, P., Desouky, A., Han, L. and Kaufman, M. (1992) Lewy bodies in psychiatric patients. *International Journal of Geriatric Psychiatry*, **7**, 235–40.
5. Shulman, K.I., Tohen, M. and Satlin, A. (1992) Mania revisited, in *Recent Advances in Psychogeriatrics* (2) (ed. T. Arie), Churchill Livingstone, Edinburgh, pp 71–80.
6. Lindesay, J. (1991) Phobic disorders in the elderly. *British Journal of Psychiatry*, **159**, 531–41.
7. Kay, D.W., Beamish, P. and Roth, M. (1964) Old age mental disorders in Newcastle-upon-Tyne. *British Journal of Psychiatry*, **110**, 146–58.
8. Petry, S., Cummings, J.L., Hill, M.A. and Shapira, J. (1989) Personality alterations in dementia of the Alzheimer type: a three-year follow-up study. *Journal of Geriatric Psychiatry and Neurology*, **2**, 203–7.
9. Kroessler, D. (1990) Personality disorder in the elderly. *Hospital and Community Psychiatry*, **41**, 1325–9.
10. Vestal, R.E., McGuire, E.A., Tobin, J.D. *et al.* (1977) Ageing and ethanol metabolism. *Clinical Pharmacology and Therapeutics*, **21**, 343–54.
11. Edwards, G., Hawker, A., Hensman, C. *et al.* (1973) Alcoholics known or unknown to agencies: epidemiological studies in a London suburb. *British Journal of Psychiatry*, **123**, 169.
12. Seymour, J. and Wattis, J.P. (1992) Alcohol abuse in the elderly. *Reviews in Clinical Gerontology*, **2**, 141–50.

4

Mood disorder: depression and mania

The feeling of depression is something we have all experienced. The 'Monday morning' feeling is familiar to most of us. When feelings of depression, often mixed with anxiety, pervade our lives, then there is something wrong that may be helped medically or psychologically. Because depression is a more or less universal experience, the dividing line between normal experience and the milder forms of depressive disorder is difficult to define. Figures for the prevalence of milder forms of depression vary widely.

4.1 CLASSIFICATION

Psychiatrists vary in the way they classify different types of depression and how they relate one type of depression to others [1]. ICD10 [2] (see Chapter 3) groups all mood disorders together under seven main categories (see Table 4.1).

Each category is subdivided according to severity (mild, moderate, severe) and the presence or absence of psychotic symptoms (hallucinations or delusions). There is also provision to register the presence or absence of 'somatic symptoms' including the loss of the capacity to experience pleasure (anhedonia), mood worse in the morning and early morning wakening.

This descriptive approach is much more logical than that of the previous edition of the International Classification of Diseases (ICD9) but unfortunately it generates over 30 categories for depression and at least eight for elevated mood!

Table 4.1 Main ICD10 categories for mood disorder

F30	Manic episode
F31	Bipolar affective disorder (includes recurrent mania)
F32	Depressive episode
F33	Recurrent depressive disorder
F34	Persistent mood (affective) disorder
F38	Other mood disorder
F39	Unspecified mood disorder

4.1.1 A practical approach

For our purposes, a description of the patient's condition and an estimation of the relative importance of early learning, current psycho-social stress, genetic endowment and biological features seem of more practical use. The practical question is not whether a person's depression should be treated biochemically, socially or psychologically but what mixture of these approaches is appropriate to the individual. The following description of categories covers the main types of depression found in old age, and corresponding ICD10 terms are given for those who wish to read fuller descriptions.

4.1.2 Dysthymia (F34.1)

This has largely replaced the term 'depressive neurosis' used in the first edition of this book. It describes people whose outlook in life is persistently depressed, but whose depression is not severe enough or clear-cut in starting and ending to merit the diagnosis of depressive episode. Anxiety is often prominent. The roots of this kind of problem are probably based more in life experience rather than in genetically determined biochemical change. Dysthymia may be a life-long problem or may be seen for the first time in response to the stresses of late life, sometimes in the aftermath of a discrete depressive episode.

4.1.3 Depressive episodes (ICD10; F32, F33)

These are characterized by depressed mood, loss of interest and enjoyment, reduced energy, increased fatiguability and reduced activity, concentration and self-esteem (often coupled with a negative evaluation of past and future). Ideas of guilt, unworthiness and ill health may reach delusional intensity. Diminished appetite and sex-drive are often found and there may be ideas that life is not worth living sometimes proceeding to self-harm or suicide. In severe forms, energy may be so reduced that the patient is immobile and uncommunicative (depressive stupor). As well as delusions, people with **psychotic** depression may hear voices saying bad things about them or accusing them of doing evil, or perceive unpleasant smells sometimes attributed to physical illness. At the most severe end of the spectrum, sufferers may neglect basic needs and have delusions that they are dead or that their bodies or bowels are rotting away ('nihilistic delusions'). An individual **depressive episode** (F32) is rare in old age; more usually the pattern is of **recurrent depressive disorder** (F33).

As patients lapse into or recover from such a state, they may go through a period of increased anxiety, sometimes with profoundly histrionic behaviour such as undressing in public or constantly demanding attention and reassurance. Depression often emphasizes the worst aspects of personality and helpers have to beware of the trap of relatives who say 'she's always been like this' when they really mean she has always had these tendencies to, for example, excessive dependency, but these have worsened recently. For a classical research-based description of depressive illness in old people, see Post [3].

4.1.4 'Reactive depression'

This term has been used to define a group of depressions which are a reaction to life circumstances and recover when these improve. In old age, severe depressive illness is not infrequently a reaction to bereavement, and may require medical as well as psychological treatment before it resolves. 'Reactivity of mood' has also been used to describe the capability of some less severely depressed patients to 'cheer up' when in company, meeting the grandchildren, etc. Because of its varied usage, some would like to exclude **reactive depression** as a diagnostic term although a modified version of the concept is still retained in ICD10 as **brief or prolonged depressive reaction** (F43.20 or F43.21).

4.1.5 'Pervasive depression'

This concept has been used by epidemiologists to describe depression of a severity or type likely to warrant medical or psychological intervention. It would include all those we have grouped under depressive episode and a proportion of those who might be labelled dysthymic.

4.2 PREVALENCE

Epidemiological studies are notoriously difficult to conduct in psychiatry, especially when older people are included [4]. Depressive disorders in the community are no more common in old age though first psychiatric admissions for depression increase in old age, probably because of severity, social factors and physical illness. Milder depressions peak before 40 years of age, more severe disorders later. Women outnumber men in all depressive diagnoses earlier in life but by the age of 65 years, the prevalence is more or less equal. A fair estimate of overall prevalence rates over 65 is about two to three per cent for severe depressions and 10 to 14 per cent for 'pervasive depressions'. Studies which have looked for symptoms associated with depression rather than a psychiatric diagnosis show a progressive increase of symptoms with increasing age in the over-20-year-old adult. When depressive symptoms have been used as screening criteria to identify patients who may be suffering from pervasive depression, as many as 40 per cent of the elderly have been found to have these symptoms. Several explanations for this are possible. One might be that transitory depressive phenomena which would not satisfy diagnostic criteria for depressive disorder are commoner in old age. Another might be that psychiatrists are more reluctant to make a diagnosis of depressive disorder with increasing age; yet another that certain physical signs and symptoms in old age might be mistakenly seen as signs of physical illness rather than depression.

4.3 CAUSES

4.3.1 Genetic susceptibility and life events

The inheritance of a tendency towards depressive episodes and mania is well documented. Generally, the later the onset of a disorder, the less important are genetic factors. A link between the onset of severe depression in old age and major life events such as bereavement has been clearly demonstrated [5]. One theory that has been put forward to explain why people with an inherited tendency develop a depressive episode in response to some stresses and not to others is that the predisposition is expressed in phases of biochemical vulnerability (Figure 4.1).

Quite a severe life event might be weathered at point 1, a major trauma might be needed to initiate a depressive attack at point 2 but at point 3 a minor trauma might suffice. This model also explains why anti-depressant therapy often has to be continued for months or years but can then sometimes be withdrawn without a recurrence of depression, at least in the short term. Between points 2 and 4 in the figure, once the depressive episode had started, biochemical treatment might be needed to suppress the symptoms. Once point 4 is reached, the treatment is no longer needed. This model would allow for different periodicity in different sufferers and for biochemically mediated increasing frequency of vulnerable periods with increasing age. Although theoretically attractive, it is not easy to prove or disprove this model experimentally.

4.3.2 Biochemical theories

Various brain amines, notably noradrenaline (NA) and serotonin (5-hydroxytriptamine) and their metabolic products have been found to be depleted in the brains of patients who have died while severely depressed. Studies on urine and cerebrospinal fluid have also shown decreased metabolites of these neurotransmitters although there has been debate about the significance of these findings. The interaction of different neurotransmitter systems has resulted in debate as to whether the primary deficiency is of NA or serotonin. A deficiency of dopamine (DA), another brain amine, is associated with Parkinson's disease, relatively common in old age and fre-

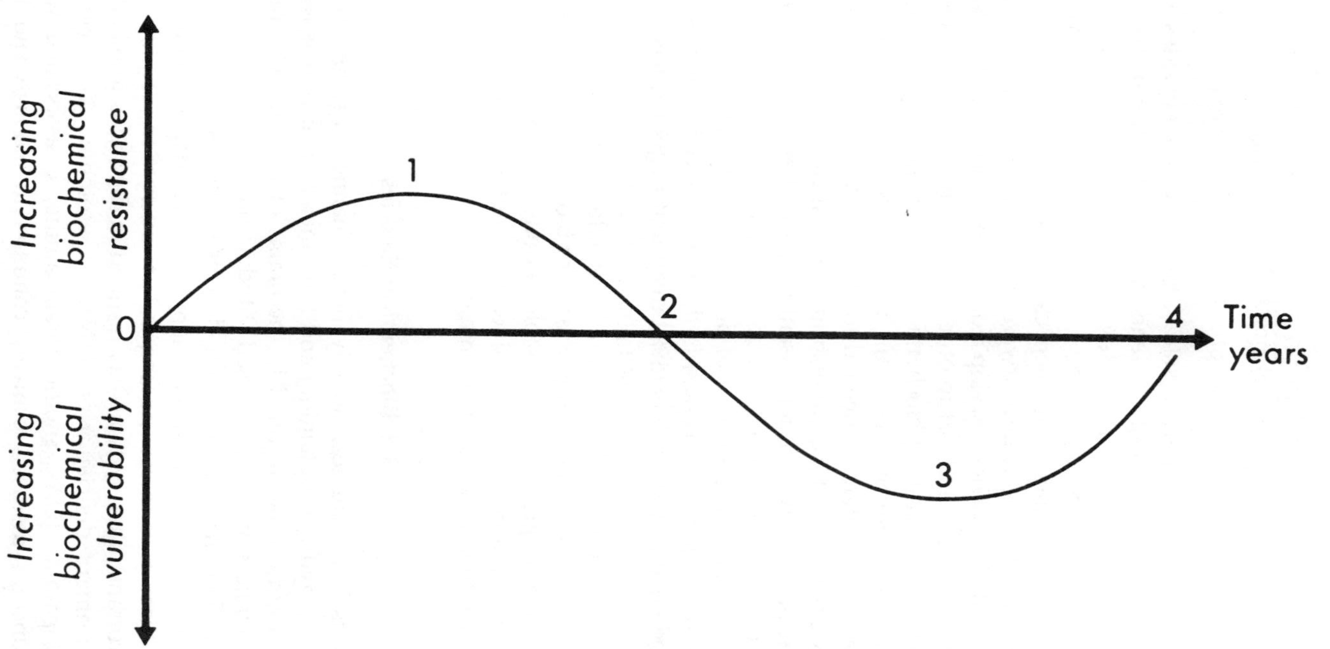

Figure 4.1 Phases of vulnerability to depression.

quently associated with depressed mood. Drugs which decrease brain amines (e.g. reserpine) produce depressed mood and at least some of the drugs used to treat depression work by enhancing the availability of amines at brain-receptor sites. A whole new group of anti-depressants, the serotonin specific reuptake inhibitors (SSRIs – see Chapter 9) has been successfully developed to target the symptoms of depression without some of the unwanted effects of earlier drugs. Interesting biochemical findings in normal ageing are small decreases in brain amines and an increase in blood platelet mono-amine oxidase activity. Mono-amine oxidases are concerned with the breakdown of transmitters such as NA and serotonin. These changes, superimposed on the phases of vulnerability already postulated in Figure 4.1, might explain the clinically observed tendency to increasing frequency of depression as people with recurrent depressive disorder grow older. The effect of biochemical ageing could be expressed on this model by an upward shift of the horizontal axis, increasing the vulnerable periods.

A subgroup of elderly depressed patients has been found in neurophysiological [6] and computerized axial tomography (CAT scan) [7, 8] studies with findings mid-way between those of normal controls and demented patients. They do not generally go on to develop dementia but they may represent a subgroup of elderly depressed patients who have brain damage underlying their depression. Depression following stroke may be significantly related to the location of the lesion on CAT scan [9], though this is disputed.

4.3.3 Bereavement

Following bereavement, four components of normal grief have been described in our society [10]. An initial stage of numbness is followed by a period of restlessness and pining. A time of anger comes next, sometimes directed at helping professionals, sometimes at the deceased or sometimes inwardly with accompanying guilt. During this phase, a degree of social withdrawal and mild depression of mood is normal but sometimes the depression may go 'out of control' and the sufferer then exhibits all the features of a severe depressive episode, including a particularly high risk of suicide. This is not the only cause of increased mortality in bereaved people. In men especially, the death rate from physical illness in the year following bereavement increases beyond chance expectation and three-quarters of these deaths are due to heart problems. People really do seem to die of a 'broken heart'. Somatic anxiety symptoms, headache and digestive upsets, also commonly occur in bereavement. The final phase of normal grieving is a resolution and adaptation to life without the dead person. The process of grieving is individual and to some extent culturally determined [11]. The components described above can merge one with another, and need not be in the order described. Recently bereaved people are a high-risk group who merit special attention and help, if necessary, to enable them to work through their feelings of depression and bereavement and to enable early detection and treatment of any depression which seems not to be self-limiting. We have come across a group of elderly depressed bereaved people who find it hard to talk about, or show much apparent emotion concerning, their lost spouse. Persistent bereavement work may be necessary to unlock this stubborn kind of grief.

A special kind of grief can be experienced by the spouses or children of people with dementia. The person they love is sometimes so diminished and changed by the disease that the relative feels they have somehow 'lost' the demented person. This 'living bereavement' often occurs at a time when the relative is having to provide extra personal care to the sufferer, making it especially hard to cope with.

4.3.4 Social factors

Severe life events such as bereavement, major social difficulties and poor health act as provoking factors for depressive illness in old people. Old people without a close, confiding relationship are especially vulnerable to the operation of such provoking factors [5].

4.3.5 Physical health

The same research has demonstrated a close relationship between continued physical ill-health or recurrent episodes of physical illness and persistent or relapsing depressive episodes.

4.3.6 Psychological factors

A psychological model of depression was developed by Seligman [12]. He showed, through animal experiments, that where outcome was made independent of behavioural response, animals lapsed into a state of 'learned helplessness' which, he argued, was analogous to the human experience of depression. He also demonstrated depletion of noradrenaline in the brains of experimental animals, providing a tenuous link between psychological and biochemical theories. The learned helplessness was very difficult to overcome once it had been induced although, if the animal was repeatedly shown that its response did make some difference, it did gradually recover. The relevance to old people is that they, too, are subject to unpleasant events, over some of which they have little control. Compulsory retirement is usual in the UK, however good people are at their work and however much they may wish to continue, though it has now been made illegal in some states in the USA on grounds of 'ageism'. Physical disabilities may accumulate despite efforts to keep fit. Learned helplessness provides one explanation for the remarkable association of depression with physical illness in old age. Old friends may seem to die off at an alarming rate, providing a link between the learned-helplessness theory, bereavement and depression. Seligman's theory has been reformulated [13] to derive treatment strategies that include increasing the patient's skills and sense of control and increasing the patient's estimation of their own contribution to success and decreasing the tendency to self-blame. Beck [14] developed a cognitive theory of depression which gives a detailed description of a therapeutic approach and procedures to use with somebody who is depressed. Cognitive therapy emphasizes the role of the individual's evaluation of any situation in determining both mood and behaviour (see Figure 8.2). The more an individual evaluates any life situation in a negative way, the greater the risk of becoming depressed. Characteristically, the depressed person has negative views of the self, the world and the future. Therapeutic interventions are aimed at enabling the individual to evaluate life experiences more accurately, and to behave in a less depressed way which leads to reduced feelings of depression (see Case history 6.3). Cognitive therapy can be used on an individual or group basis.

Of all the psychotherapeutic approaches to depression, it has the most empirical evidence to support its efficacy.

Interpersonal interactions can help maintain depressed mood [15]. People who are depressed behave in ways that encourage other people to avoid them or to become angry (often without showing it). Other psychological formulations of depression deal with the loss of meaning in life as various roles become unavailable to the older person. To avoid or ease depression, new ways of deriving meaning have to be developed [16]. These are discussed further in Chapter 8 on psychological treatment.

4.4 PROGNOSIS

Research studies have given contrasting pictures of the prognosis of depression in old age. Some findings have suggested that just over one-third of depressed patients have a good outcome at one year, a similar proportion deteriorate or die and a smaller fraction remain unchanged [17]. More recent studies with a longer time frame and possibly more complete treatment of depressive episodes have found a relatively better prognosis with at least two-thirds of patients making a full recovery or having a further successfully treated episode [18]. We believe that a whole-person approach to depressed patients can improve prognosis. The association with physical illness and uncontrollable life events such as bereavement and admission to an institution suggest possible mediators for poor prognosis. Other factors associated with poor prognosis are duration of more than one or two years before treatment, increasing age, and severity (see Table 4.2).

Table 4.2 Factors associated with poor prognosis in depressed old people

Psychotic illness with depressive delusions
Increased duration of illness
Physical illness
Low social class (more likely to suffer severe life events)
Housing difficulties
Low income
Severe life events in the year after the initial episode

We can use these prognostic factors to develop an understanding of how to improve the management of depression in old age. Increased duration of depression may mean that, in addition to biochemical changes, the patient has also developed depressive habits and that the family and neighbours have evolved compensatory ways of behaving that tend to perpetuate the depressive behaviour, even after adequate physical treatment. The patient who has been depressed for a long time, therefore, needs not only biochemical treatment but also intervention based on a careful evaluation of psycho-social factors that may be maintaining the illness. Severity of depression may be a prognostic factor because people with severe depression are not always treated adequately. Recent popular pressure against ECT (see Chapter 9), particularly useful in severe depression with delusions or psychomotor retardation, has sometimes deterred doctors from using this treatment. Severely depressed patients are notoriously poor at taking medication regularly and so when patients are discharged home before they are completely well, they may stop taking tablets and relapse. Careful follow-up helps reduce the risk of this happening. Associated physical illness needs active treatment and review. We cannot prevent some traumatic life events, such as bereavement, for patients who have been depressed, but we can ensure that there is somebody, either friend or professional, available to support patients through such life events. Poor physical design in psychiatric units can reduce the chances of successful treatment by reducing self-esteem, opportunities for interpersonal interactions and mobility. Staff skills and attitudes are also relevant. This is discussed further in Chapter 8. Case history 4.1 is an good example of how a patient with an apparently poor prognosis can have a happy outcome with the holistic approach.

Case history 4.1:

Mrs B.R. was a 66-year-old married lady with a history of chronic depression. She had been admitted to the psychiatric unit 16 times in 14 years and had never been well for any sustained period since the age of 55 years when her mother died. After her first admission under our care she was discharged home but refused to come to day hospital and took to her bed. She had nihilistic delusions (that she had no pulse) and was readmitted. When her previous history was reviewed we found that she had always failed to take adequate doses of anti-depressants because of alleged side-effects. She also behaved in a highly dependent way and her relationship with her husband was one of mutual hostility. When she again refused to co-operate in treatment, she was put on a compulsory treatment order and given gradually increasing doses of tricyclic anti-depressant. Despite an observed improvement in her mood over several months, she said she felt no better and hostile-dependent behaviour continued. A behavioural and cognitive treatment programme was instituted and slow improvement continued. She and her husband seemed unable to appreciate this and an extremely hostile interaction continued. Marital therapy was instituted and after six months Mrs B.R. was discharged from inpatient care. Despite her attendance at day hospital while on the ward, on discharge she refused to attend further, and weekly home visits were carried out by the psychologist and a member of the ward staff. At first, the situation at home caused concern, as she took to lying in bed until lunchtime, complaining of pain. However, the nursing assistant noticed on one visit that Mrs B.R. was showing signs of arthritis in her hands (not apparent on the ward). This was treated in collaboration with the GP, and she continued to improve slowly. The final intervention, a housing transfer, which had been given medical priority, enabled her to live near one daughter and her grandchildren. This allowed her to have a meaningful and constructive family life again, and was agreed with the daughter (both the daughters had been closely involved throughout treatment). Over the months, professional support was gradually reduced, the daughters continuing to slowly rehabilitate their mother. Two years later, she remained extremely well, despite having discontinued her anti-depressant medication after one year.

This case illustrates how even severe long-term depression can be helped with a sustained and co-ordinated approach to treatment. If any of the interventions (medical, psychological and social) had been mistimed, inappropriately carried out, or missed completely, this old person might have continued to relapse and to live an unhappy and unfulfilled life.

The lesser side-effects and lower toxicity of the newer anti-depressants also offer increased hope for patients who are unable to tolerate the side-effects of the conventional tricyclics. Combination therapy with lithium helps in some cases, as does the prophylactic use of lithium or anti-depressants in patients with recurrent depressive disorder.

4.5 MANAGEMENT

4.5.1 Assessment

The proper assessment of a depressed old person involves much more than just making a diagnosis. Figure 4.2 summarizes the interactive model of depression outlined in this chapter.

Periodic phases of vulnerability to depression, genetically determined and biochemically mediated, are the basis of severe recurrent depressive disorder. However, a severe depressive

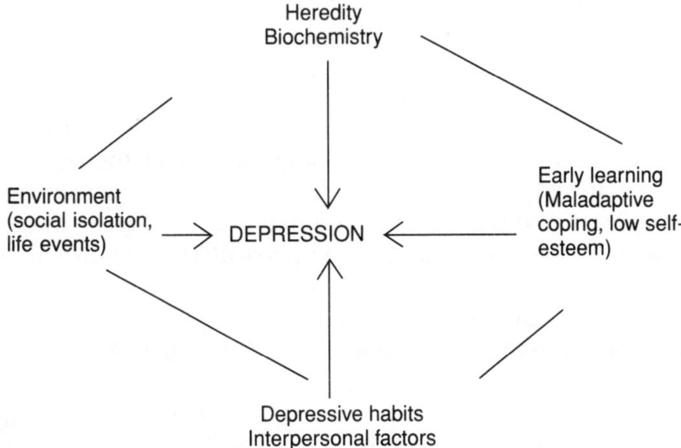

Figure 4.2 Factors contributing to causing and maintaining depression.

episode can also arise *de novo* in old age in response to a major stress such as bereavement. People who have evolved maladaptive styles of coping with life at an early age, especially those who are rigid, insecure or over-anxious, may be more susceptible to depressive episodes and dysthymia in old age. All depressions may be complicated by depressive habits of behaviour and the way that other people react to these. Assessment is not, therefore, a question of just assigning a depression to a particular ICD10 category but of determining the balance of initiating and maintaining causes from the selection in Figure 4.2.

(a) History

This should be obtained from an independent informant as well as the patient. The time-course of the illness should be ascertained as well as its severity and how far it is threatening life by self-neglect or suicidal intent. The patient's previous personality and any previous episodes of affective disorder should be investigated. A family history of affective disorder should be sought. Possible precipitating or maintaining factors in the environment (e.g. bereavement, ill-health or other 'loss' events) should be explored. A special note should be made of any alteration in behaviour of friends and relatives in response to the patient's illness, as this may have to be dealt with as part of the patient's treatment.

(b) Mental state

The patient's cleanliness and general appearance and behaviour should be noted. If she lives alone, a tour of the house may reveal an empty larder and other signs of recent self-neglect. One depressed old lady had the previous few weeks meals-on-wheels' deliveries stacked in a cupboard! The patient will often appear depressed but sometimes all her energy will be invested in hypochondriacal or persecutory complaints and she may then not admit to feeling depressed. Sleep disturbance, especially early morning wakening and diurnal variation of mood (usually feeling worse in the morning), are often found, especially in the more severe depressive episodes. Loss of the ability to take pleasure in anything (anhedonia) and loss of drive are other common findings. Thoughts are often preoccupied with ideas of poverty, guilt or illness and these worries may reach delusional intensity. The speed of thought and talk may be profoundly slowed. This depressive retardation may co-exist with agitation, a very uncomfortable state of affairs for the patient. Retardation is also one of the factors that can produce apparent cognitive impairment. If given plenty of time, the retarded patient may improve her performance on cognitive tests. *Severe* cognitive impairment in a depressive episode (sometimes called 'depressive pseudo-dementia') is correlated with an increased likelihood that the patient will develop true dementia if followed up for long enough, even though the acute episode apparently responds well to treatment.

Psychomotor slowing is also a feature of the 'subcortical' syndrome (see Chapter 5) and its presence should always lead to consideration of special investigations such as tests for vitamin B12 and thyroid deficiency. In difficult cases, perhaps the best test of whether cognitive impairment is secondary to depression is to treat the depression, preferably with an anti-depressant devoid of anti-cholinergic action, and see if cognitive function and behaviour improve. It should also never be forgotten that dementia confers no immunity to depression and indeed early dementia is often associated with depressed mood. In these cases, cautious use of a non-anti-cholinergic anti-depressant is fully justified.

(c) Physical examination

Depressed mood is associated with physical illness in old age. Stroke, perhaps especially with lesions in the frontal or occipito-parietal regions, is associated with depressed mood [9]. Depression may be the first presentation of a hidden neoplasm. There are particularly strong relationships between depression and cardiovascular disease, Parkinsonism, metabolic upsets, especially electrolyte imbalance, thyroid deficiency and vitamin B12 deficiency. Relevant physical examination and appropriate biochemical and haematological investigations are therefore useful in all cases and mandatory where there is no response to adequate anti-depressant treatment.

4.5.2 Problem formulation

Having assembled the data, it is essential to formulate the problems and prepare a management plan. All factors should be taken into account and a problem list is an effective way of doing this. A particularly important decision is whether the patient should be treated at home or in hospital and social circumstances as well as severity of illness and suicide risk are important in this decision. The following case histories illustrate some of the important points in the management of depression. More details of physical and psychological treatments for depression are given in Chapters 8 and 9.

Case history 4.2:

A 72-year-old married women had a history of two previous severe depressive episodes, the last only in the previous year. She lost interest in her husband and house over a period of a few weeks and became extremely agitated. Her relatives were distressed and feared she might take an overdose. The general practitioner was called in and the psychiatrist was consulted. The old lady confided in him that, as a result of a liaison with a soldier during the war, she believed that she had contracted venereal disease and this was allegedly ruining her husband and daughter (both perfectly healthy people). This depressive delusion was held in the face of all evidence to the contrary. Eventually she accepted inpatient treatment with ECT, although she was convinced it would not do any good. She made a full recovery and has remained well on lithium therapy. Her depressive episode had no obvious precipitant and presented in a straightforward way, which is relatively unusual in elderly people.

Case history 4.3:

This 82-year-old lady was gradually losing her sight. She came from Germany and had successfully coped with the Second World War and its aftermath, despite living in the

Communist-occupied zone. She had subsequently escaped to England with her husband, where she enjoyed an active life, bringing up her family and teaching German and continental cookery. She found the restrictions of old age, especially her deteriorating sight, extremely difficult to cope with and began to respond by spending a lot of her time in bed. She took a small overdose of the sleeping tablet, nitrazepam and the general practitioner referred her for a psychiatric opinion. She had none of the features of severe depression, although her mother had, in fact, committed suicide following the Second World War. The diagnosis was of a mild depressive episode (F32.0) precipitated and maintained by deteriorating eyesight and restricted lifestyle. She was treated at home with twelve weekly sessions of cognitive psychotherapy. She made an excellent response, despite some early problems, gradually resuming previous activities and learning to cope with her poor eyesight which was subsequently corrected by a cataract operation.

Case history 4.4:

A widow in her seventies became depressed when her daughter's marriage broke up and the daughter and grand-daughter moved into her small flat. She could not cope and went to her general practitioner, who prescribed imipramine. Unfortunately, an interaction between this and the beta-adrenergic blocking drug she was using caused her blood pressure to drop precipitously whenever she stood up. Hospital admission was needed to treat this. Once the daughter and grand-daughter were found alternative accommodation nearby, her depression lifted and she did not need drugs.

These case histories illustrate the variety of different presentations of depression in old age and the variety of approaches needed to cope with them. A true multi-disciplinary approach offers the best hope for the old person. Figure 4.3 is a flow

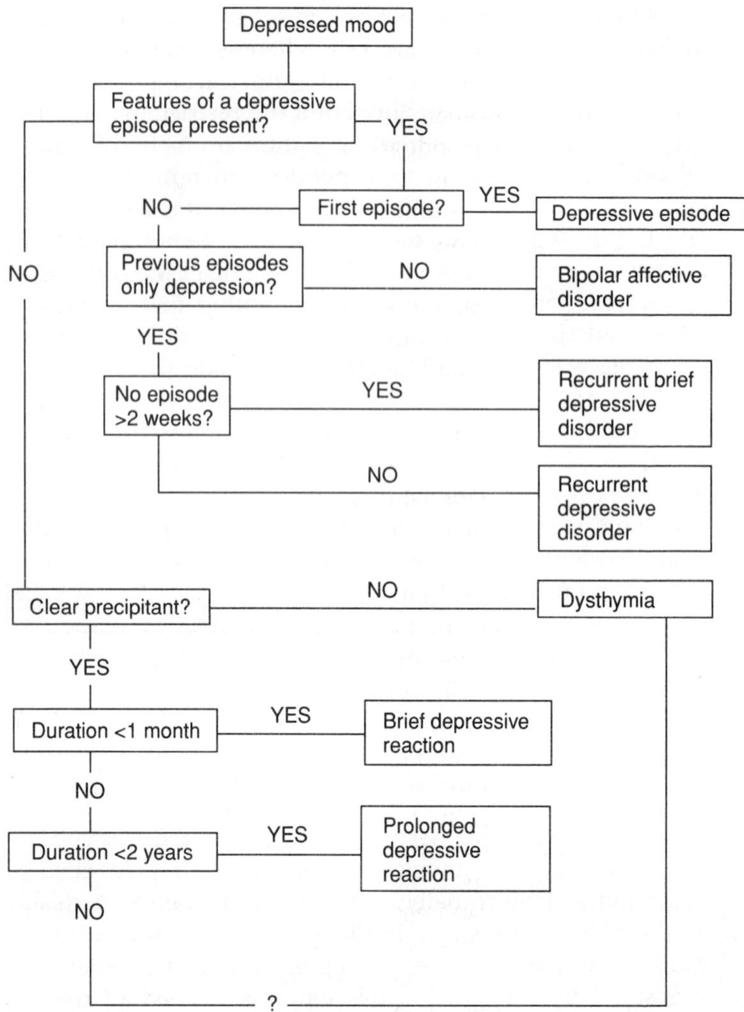

Figure 4.3 Flow chart of the diagnosis of a patient with depressed mood according to simplified ICD10 criteria.

chart to help in the diagnosis of depression in old age. It should not be used by itself to plan management. Many depressed patients will require a mixture of physical treatment and psychological and social help to give them the best chance of recovery.

The proportion of these different ingredients to the management plan will, of course, vary from patient to patient as Case histories 4.1 to 4.4 demonstrate. The timing of interventions is also crucial. Thus, a woman with marital problems and a severe psychotic depressive episode might require inpatient treatment with ECT followed by marital therapy. To put the marital therapy first could waste time in unsuccessful efforts, with the patient not in a state to respond. To ignore the marital problem after ECT would be to make full recovery less likely and relapse more probable. Management should be planned as a problem-solving exercise with the problems arranged according to the order in which they should be tackled.

4.5.3 Prevention

Improving family relationships and the capacity to make meaningful choices in later life should protect some old people against depression, as should the prompt diagnosis and effective treatment of physical illness. Counselling for people with long-term illness about the nature of their illness and ways to overcome disability helps restore choices and some feeling of control. Spiritual and religious understanding of life problems can help people understand the meaning of threatening life events. Extra financial support for people with long-standing disability enhances control and enables better coping strategies. People who are recently bereaved should be offered tactful emotional and practical support and, if necessary, formal counselling. As well as reducing the incidence of depressive episodes, this might also help to reduce the excessive mortality from physical, especially cardiovascular, problems. The routine prescription of anti-depressants to bereaved people should be avoided; the older tricyclics may increase the risk of cardiovascular deaths and anti-depressants like tranquillizers may interfere with normal grieving. Once depression has occurred, sustained treatment with anti-depressants and/or lithium may be needed to prevent recurrence. Psychotherapeutic approaches (e.g. cognitive therapy, brief psychotherapy, bereavement counselling) may be needed to improve the person's self-image and problem-solving ability which, in turn, may reduce the likelihood of relapse. Day-hospital treatment can be an alternative to admission or can enable early discharge from inpatient treatment. Continuing Day Centre support can help those who are lonely and, if threatening life events occur, prompt intervention can reduce the risk of repeated depression. Formal family therapy and other work with the family can help re-establish a healthy role for the sufferer in home life. These are all common-sense approaches. It is difficult to verify their effectiveness experimentally (except for drug-maintenance therapy) but case-studies do suggest that they are effective and worthwhile in reducing recurrence of depression.

4.6 MANIA/HYPOMANIA (ICD10; F30) AND BIPOLAR AFFECTIVE DISORDER (F31)

Mania and hypomania are much less common than recurrent depressive disorder in late life and are rarely seen except in the context of previous episodes of depressive disorder. Hypomania is basically a milder version of mania and the two terms are used interchangeably here. A fair proportion of people with recurrent depressive illness develop mania or hypomania for the first time in late life and a significant number have organic brain damage (not dementia) [19]. Over-activity without cognitive impairment is the cardinal clinical feature. The elation and infectious good humour of the younger hypomanic may be replaced by irritability and querulousness, though recent research has suggested that the phenomenology of mania in old people is very similar to that in younger people. Grandiose ideas and delusions are entertained, sometimes with a mixture of persecutory ideas. Alcohol abuse with frontal-lobe impairment may mimic mania although excessive drinking may also sometimes be symptomatic of mania. The association between alcoholic brain damage and late-onset mania is not clear (see Case history 4.5). There is usually no cognitive impairment though this may have to be inferred indirectly as the patient may not co-operate with detailed mental state examination. Mixed-mood states with hypomanic over-activity but depressive ideas also occur. The patient is often extremely difficult to help and inpatient treatment, often under a compulsory order, is usually necessary. Response to initial treatment with neuroleptics is usually good (zuclopenthixol may be especially useful). Lithium can also be used in the acute phase though there is some delay in the onset of its anti-manic action. If the affective illness is recurrent, with more than one episode every few years, then continuing lithium therapy is appropriate. The use of lithium in old people demands careful monitoring because of the risks of toxicity but the excellent results fully justify the risk. Environmental and family factors, especially those associated with failure to continue medication, such as living alone, must be considered. A patient who has been manic for a long time needs an extended period of stability in

Case history 4.5:

Mr S.V. was 66 years old when he first came to our notice. He was grossly over-active and had (single-handedly) demolished part of his house as a preliminary to extensions he never carried out. He had purchased a number of luxury items, including a 'state of the art' microwave oven which he was using as a cupboard. He was hardly sleeping, drinking excessively and amazingly full of energy. He had to be admitted to hospital on Section 3 (s.3) of the Mental Health Act (MHA) and required, for his age, prodigious doses of zuclopenthixol and lithium before his mania came under control. After discharge he was maintained under close supervision in the day hospital where the neuroleptics were gradually withdrawn over a period of about a year and lithium was maintained. He was discharged to a Day Centre with out-patient clinic follow-up. He was regarded as a capable helper as well as a client in the Day Centre. On a trip out he was noted to drink ten pints of beer. Soon, he was once more grandiose and over-active with schemes to get social security benefits on behalf of 'single-parent mothers' and to reintroduce corporal punishment and hanging. He again had to be admitted to hospital, initially informally but then on s.3 after he absconded and created a disturbance at a relative's house. His illness again came under control with firm but sympathetic nursing care to ensure (among other things) that he took his prescribed medication.

hospital and particularly careful rehabilitation if relapse is to be avoided.

REFERENCES

1. Kendell, R.E. (1976) The classification of depression: a review of contemporary confusion. *British Journal of Psychiatry*, **129**, 15–28.
2. World Health Organization (1992) *The ICD10 classification of mental and behavioural disorders: clinical descriptions and diagnostic guidelines.* World Health Organization, Geneva.
3. Post, F. (1982) Functional disorders, in *The Psychiatry of Late Life*, (eds R. Levy and F. Post), Blackwell Scientific Publications, London.
4. Gurland, B.J. (1976) The comparative frequency of depression in various age groups. *Journal of Gerontology*, **31**, 283–92.
5. Murphy, E. (1982) The social origins of depression in old age. *British Journal of Psychiatry*, **141**, 135–42.
6. Hendrickson, E., Levy, R. and Post, F. (1979) Averaged evoked potentials in relation to the cognitive and affective state of elderly patients. *British Journal of Psychiatry*, **134**, 494–500.
7. Jacoby, R., Levy, R. and Bird, J.M. (1981) Computed tomography and the outcome of affective disorder: a follow-up study of elderly patients. *British Journal of Psychiatry*, **139**, 288–92.
8. Jacoby, R., Dolan, R., Levy, R. and Baldy, R. (1983) Quantitative computed tomography in elderly depressed patients. *British Journal of Psychiatry*, **143**, 124–7.
9. Lipsey, J.R., Robinson, R.G., Pearlson, G.D. *et al.* (1983) Mood change following bilateral hemisphere brain injury. *British Journal of Psychiatry*, **143**, 266–73.
10. Parkes, C.M. (1986) *Bereavement: Studies of Grief in Adult Life*, Pelican, London.
11. Parkes, C.M. (1985) Bereavement. *British Journal of Psychiatry*, **146**, 11–17.
12. Seligman, M.E. (1975) *Helplessness: on Depression, Development and Death*, Freeman, San Francisco.
13. Abramson, L.Y., Seligman, M.E. and Teesdale, J.D. (1978) Learned helplessness in humans: critique and reformulation. *Journal of Abnormal Psychology*, **87**, 49–74.
14. Beck, A.T., Rush, A.S., Shaw, B.E. and Emery, G. (1989) *Cognitive Therapy of Depression*, Penguin Books, London.
15. Coyne, J.C. (1986) Towards an interactional description of depression, in *Essential Papers on Depression*, (ed. J. Coyne), New York University Press, New York.
16. Becker, E.S. (1986) Depression: a comprehensive theory, in *Essential Papers on Depression*, (ed. J. Coyne), New York University Press, New York.
17. Murphy, E. (1983) The prognosis of depression in old age. *British Journal of Psychiatry*, **142**, 111–19.

18. Baldwin, R. and Jolley, D. (1986) The prognosis of depression in old age. *British Journal of Psychiatry*, **149**, 577–83.
19. Shulman, K.I., Tohen, M. and Satlin, A. (1992) Mania revisited, in *Recent Advances in Psychogeriatrics (2)*, (ed. T. Arie), Churchill Livingstone, Edinburgh, pp 71–80.

5

Confusion

The confused patient does not usually ask for help. The general practitioner or social services are called in by worried relatives or neighbours or the confusion is noticed when the patient is admitted to hospital for some other reason. Helping the confused patient is a difficult task for a variety of reasons. Proper background knowledge to understand the causes of the patient's confusion may be lacking; the community support and institutional care services may be inadequate and the patient may not be able to co-operate fully in using those services which are available.

5.1 EPIDEMIOLOGY AND SOCIAL POLICY

This chapter deals with both transient acute confusional states (delirium) and the more chronic states generally called dementia. Because delirium is transient and often associated with severe physical illness, its exact prevalence is hard to measure and it is excluded from this section of the chapter.

5.1.1 Prevalence

The overall prevalence rate for dementia in the over-65s is around ten per cent rising from two per cent of the 65–69-year age group to around 20 per cent of over-85-year-old people [1]. Since the first edition of this book epidemiological studies have been repeated in many settings and there is a striking similarity between the rates found in different studies and especially in the steep rise with increasing age. The oldest groups have more physical and social handicaps and are more likely to need continuing institutional care. Overall survival of old people with dementia has increased over the last 25 years or so [2]. The implication of this and of the decreasing ratio of middle-aged to elderly people is that more community care and more institutional care will be needed over the next 20 years.

5.1.2 Guidelines

The Health Advisory Service report *The Rising Tide* [3] and, more recently, a joint publication by the Royal Colleges of Physicians and Psychiatrists in 1989 [4] set out basic requirements for providing psychiatric services to old people and, in the latter case, for training doctors in the specialty.

5.1.3 Continuing care and restructuring of the NHS

In the radical restructuring of the British National Health Service, funds for continuing care have largely been shifted into the private sector but this has been based on political dogma rather than any certainty that this is a better or even a cheaper way of caring. Between 1985 and April 1993 funds were available in the UK through the social security system for those going into private residential or nursing-home care. This produced a boom in private provision at the public's expense. The government decided to put a limit on this funding by channelling it through local social services authorities who have been expected to assess and pay for new entrants into residential and nursing-home care since April 1993, on a **means-tested** basis. There are concerns that this will be funded insufficiently, that local authorities will introduce bureaucratic delays and that there will be ambiguity in both social services and health authorities being responsible for purchasing continuing care, especially since one will be means tested and one will be free at the point of use.

5.1.4 Personal needs of carers and patients

In addition to the vast increase in epidemiological and basic scientific research, there has been a welcome increase in research into the human aspects of dementia with an increasing literature on the needs of carers [5] and even an attempt to look at the needs of demented people themselves [6].

The way in which we treat old people suffering from mental illness and dementia has improved in the period since the first edition of this book, but remains a major social scandal in the face of our spending in other areas. The shift towards a more market-oriented consumer society will not in itself help this group of people who are unable to stand up for their own needs; and it increases rather than decreases the responsibility of professionals working in the field to act as advocates for the needs of old people with dementia.

5.1.5 Euthanasia

After visiting some old people's homes or long-stay wards for demented patients, colleagues sometimes ask whether euthanasia would not be a better solution, in view of the poor 'quality of life' of the old people. Quite apart from the moral question of whether we have the right to terminate our own or anybody else's life, the practical question of why quality of life is poor has to be examined. Demented people are far more dependent on their environment than young people or than well old people. When nurse-staffing levels are sometimes well below recommended levels, when occupational-therapy services on the wards are virtually non-existent and when the wards themselves are sometimes badly designed relics in remote Victorian asylums, it is not surprising if quality of life is not good. The shift to well-staffed, well-designed health-service units located in the local community may now never be completed in the UK because resources have been moved to the private sector. Nor are things necessarily always better in the private homes. Although they tend to be smaller than the old asylums, there is a trend to increasing size, dictated by the economies of scale. The private homes also tend to cluster where there are large, relatively cheap houses with sympathetic local planning authorities so that there are whole areas of the large cities left without a local residential or nursing home for old people, increasing the isolation of residents who may be placed many miles from their families. Despite the fact that two-thirds of people in residential or nursing-home care suffer from dementia, staff are often inadequately trained to ensure the best quality of life for these people. Detailed knowledge now exists of how to improve and measure quality of life for demented people [7, 8] so that there is little excuse for continuing to provide poor services.

One danger of the euthanasia argument is that it is cheaper to allow old people to die than to provide adequate community services or nursing facilities. We are in danger of falling into the same trap as our ancestors by regarding old people, especially those with dementia, as less than human in much the same way that they regarded slaves as disposable personal property. In the following sections we intend to show that not all confusion in old people is due to dementia but, equally important, that when dementia is present the defeatist view that 'nothing can be done' is based on ignorance. By provision of appropriate services and training to develop appropriate skills, the quality of life of the majority of demented old people can be vastly improved.

5.2 CAUSES OF CONFUSION

5.2.1 Delirium/acute confusional states (ICD10; F05)

The term delirium has recently come back into widespread use to describe a syndrome in which there is disturbance of consciousness and attention with associated problems with memory, behaviour and the sleep-wake cycle, often accompanied by perceptual distortions (illusions) or frank hallucinations. The term **acute confusional state** is used as a synonym. Old people, especially if they are already suffering from mild dementia, are particularly prone to develop delirium. Its hallmark is sudden onset. The patient's behaviour is often erratic and bizarre and level of awareness of the environment is diminished and fluctuates, often being worse at night. The effect is of perplexity or fear and thoughts and talk are incoherent. Perceptual misinterpretations and hallucinations, especially visual, are common and may produce violent behaviour. Attention and concentration are inhibited and cognitive function is impaired. The patient may be hyperactive or hypoactive. Not surprisingly, the hypoactive cases are less likely to be noticed!

Provided the cause, which is usually physical illness, is detected and responds to treatment, prognosis for recovery of the mental state is good. The time-course of delirium is variable depending on the underlying cause, varying from a few hours

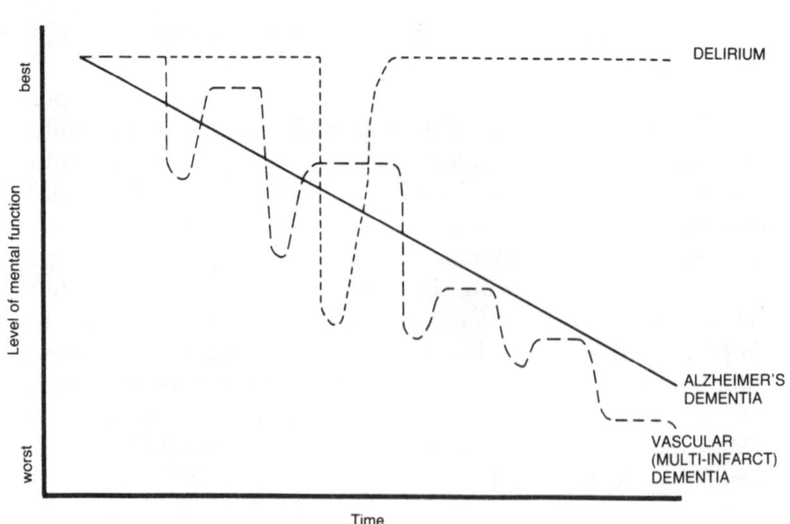

Figure 5.1 Time-course of different causes of confusion.

or days with an acute infection to weeks or even months with metabolic upset such as chronic liver disease. It is summarized in Figure 5.1. Probably because of better treatment of the underlying illness, only about a tenth of the people admitted to hospital with delirium now die before six months have elapsed, though over a third are dead at two-year follow-up, a proportion intermediate between that of those suffering from functional illness and those suffering from dementia [9]. Heart failure and infections, especially of the chest and the urinary tract, are probably the commonest causes of delirium in old age. Prescribed drugs are sometimes responsible. Long-acting benzodiazepines and drugs with marked anti-cholinergic effects such as some anti-Parkinsonian drugs and anti-depressants are among the greatest offenders. Other conditions which can contribute to delirium are summarized in Table 5.1.

Thiamine deficiency is classically associated with alcoholism and causes a delirium called Wernicke's encephalopathy, characterized by confusion, ataxia and ophthalmoplegia. This deficiency may be followed by the permanent loss of short-term memory and confabulation (Korsakoff's psychosis). Thiamine deficiency has also been implicated as a possible cause of pro-

Table 5.1 Some causes of delirium

Severe infection	**Systems failure**
chest	cardiac
urine	renal
	hepatic
Metabolic	respiratory embarrassment
diabetes	
thyroid	**Dehydration**
B12	
thiamine	**Intra-cranial**
	stroke
Drugs and toxins	subdural haematoma
carbon monoxide	other space-occupying lesions
alcohol	
anti-cholinergic drugs	**Depressive illness**
benzodiazepines	

(see also Table 2.9 for a fuller list of confusion-inducing drugs)
In those otherwise predisposed by dementia add:
change of environment
constipation
minor infection
pain

longed post-operative confusion in elderly patients presenting with fractured neck of femur. Though this finding has been disputed, it is worth considering thiamine supplements in all acutely ill old people, especially those who may have been taking a poor diet or abusing alcohol. In patients who are already suffering from dementia, a relatively trivial infection, constipation or a change of environment may be sufficient to precipitate an acute worsening of confusion (F05.1). The 'reflex diagnosis' of dementia is the greatest enemy of the acutely confused patient and if the onset of confusion is known to be sudden or if it is unknown, then a thorough medical evaluation, including a drug history and physical examination, is vital. Because of the patient's erratic behaviour and unreliability in taking medication, initial management is usually best in hospital. In most cases, the degree of physical illness will necessitate admission under the care of a physician, although less ill patients can sometimes be managed on an acute psychiatric ward for old people provided it is on a site with ready access to investigational facilities and medical help. Treatment of the underlying physical illness should be supplemented by appropriate nursing care and general management which may include the use of neuroleptics such as haloperidol, zuclopenthixol or thioridazine, though there is always a risk of increasing confusion by sedative or anti-cholinergic drugs. Management will be discussed in more detail later in this chapter.

5.2.2 Dementia in Alzheimer's disease (AD, ICD10; F0.1)

This disease is responsible for at least half of the cases of dementia that occur in old age. Women appear to be slightly more likely to be affected than men, even allowing for the greater proportion of women in the elderly population.

(a) Clinical

AD has an insidious onset with a gradual decline in the mental state (Figure 5.1). Memory difficulties, especially problems in encoding new memories, are usually the first symptoms to be noticed, though indecision and 'vagueness' are also often described. Often memory problems are attributed at first to absent-mindedness or old age. The onset is so gradual that even a close relative living with the sufferer finds it difficult to put a date on when the patient was last quite normal. In the early stages, previous personality may strongly influence the presentation. The patient with a tendency to be suspicious of others may upset carers by accusing them of stealing misplaced items. The patient with a tendency to dependency may react to these early changes by becoming extremely dependent on relatives, especially if family patterns of behaviour encourage this. Mood disturbance is not, in itself, a feature of AD, though it may be found in 15–30 per cent of patients. The patient usually lacks insight and, as the disease progresses, behaviour may become more erratic. Disorientation for time, place and person will also become more evident. A combination of restlessness (often worse in the evening) and topographical disorientation may cause the patient to wander off and get lost. The patient may get up in the early hours of the morning believing she must go to work or may insist on going 'home' early (even from her own house!) to prepare a meal for the 'children'. Caring relatives are particularly distressed if the sufferer fails to recognize them. Fortunately, this does not usually happen until a late stage of the disease, but it can be especially difficult for spouses, for example if an elderly husband is trying to help his wife with personal care and is pushed away by a wife who sees him as 'a strange man'. Spontaneous thought becomes increasingly limited as dementia develops and repetitive talk can be wearing for carers.

Hallucinations are not uncommon but are rarely evident, except through the indirect reporting of carers, unless there is a complicating delirium or severe auditory or visual handicap. Rarely, sufferers will find not only other people's faces but also their own faces difficult to recognize. A reflection perceived in a mirror can then give rise to worries that a stranger is in the house. The wife of one of our patients had to take down all the mirrors in the house because of this problem. As the disease progresses, apraxias may develop in skills such as dressing or washing or the motivation to perform these tasks may fade, further limiting the ability to live independently. Incontinence usually develops late in the course of the disease although it may occur earlier if complicating factors such as poor mobility, inconvenient location of the toilet or urinary-tract infection supervene. Dysphasia can lead to frustrating difficulties in communication for both patient and carers. Eventually the point is reached for those living alone where intermittent support is not enough and where admission to an old people's home or hospital for continuing care becomes necessary. Old people living with their families can often continue to live in at home for longer, especially if appropriate support services are offered. Often patients die from other causes before they reach the terminal stage of AD though the dementia often contributes to the death. Patients with AD usually lose a considerable amount of weight, regardless of nutritional intake, and an obese patient with advanced dementia is probably not suffering from AD. Neurological symptoms develop in the terminal stages of AD. By this time patients are often in hospital and may have developed contractures due to inadequate care. At this stage patients need total nursing care. Despite the severity of the patients' handicaps, those who nurse them still often find that they retain emotional responsiveness to their carers.

(b) Aetiology and pathology

The brains of patients suffering from AD are shrunken. Microscopically senile (amyloid) plaques are found in the brain in far greater numbers than in ordinary old people [10]. Neurofibrillary tangles, found in the hippocampal region of some normal old people, are increased in numbers and more widely distributed especially in earlier-onset cases of AD. There may be an accumulation of lipofuscin and granulovacuolar degeneration. Biochemical research has shown a markedly reduced level of the cholinergic marker enzyme, choline acetyl transferase, more localized in older subjects [11]. Deficiencies in other neuro-transmitters have also been found, especially in earlier onset cases, but they are not so marked as in the cholinergic system.

There is a genetic component to AD. Some family pedigrees have been established with dominant inheritance, usually in earlier onset disease, and there is a clear genetic link with Down's syndrome (trisomy 21) but the genetic contribution to the majority of cases is less clear. Relatives of patients with AD have a slightly increased risk of developing the disease. There is an interaction between environmental and genetic causes. It may well be that the pathological findings of AD are the end-result of a variety of different processes and that late-onset AD is aetiologically and genetically different from the earlier-onset type. Possible environmental factors include head injury (this may act as a 'trigger') and aluminium. Current research into the molecular biology of AD, including the composition of plaques and tangles, holds some hope for the eventual discovery of therapeutic measures. A really effective treatment is still probably a long way off and will have to be coupled with a reliable method for detecting the disease in its pre-clinical phase if maximum benefit is to be reaped.

(c) Diagnosis

The history is most important. Insidious onset and a gradual but inexorable progression are the rule. Mental state examination with evidence of memory loss and, in all but the earliest cases, evidence also of impairment in other areas of cortical function such as visuospatial dysfunction and nominal aphasia, help confirm the diagnosis. If the patient is seen early in the disease then basic screening tests to exclude metabolic causes of dementia (e.g. B12, thyroid) are indicated. Prominent headaches or focal signs require computerized axial tomography (CAT scan) to exclude space-occupying lesions. CAT scans show the typical brain-shrinkage of AD but the overlap with the normal or functionally ill population is too great for this to be of diagnostic use. Newer scanning techniques (such as Nuclear Magnetic Resonance, Single Positron Emission and Positron Emission Tomography) have little to offer in routine diagnostic use (at least in UK practice) but have value as research tools.

5.2.3 Vascular dementia (ICD10; F01)

This affects a fifth of patients with dementia and another fifth have a mixture of AD and vascular dementia. **Multi-infarct dementia** (MID, F01.1) is the commonest form. Men are more commonly affected than women and the 'young old' more than very elderly people. **Vascular dementia of acute onset** (F01.0) is similar to MID but develops rapidly after a series of strokes or, occasionally, a single large stroke. **Subcortical vascular dementia** is associated with infarcts deep in the white matter of the cerebral hemispheres where it can often be visualized by a CAT scan. There is often a history of hypertension and the clinical picture resembles AD. **Mixed cortical and subcortical vascular dementia** (F01.3) also occurs and is likely to be increasingly diagnosed with the more widespread use of CAT scans.

(a) Clinical

As its name implies, MID is associated with multiple cerebral infarcts. Onset is therefore usually sudden and the general progression stepwise (Figure 5.1). Often, there is a history of hypertension and there may be frank strokes or other signs of vascular disease. The patient characteristically retains more insight than in AD and often has depression or lability of mood, sometimes with uncontrollable outbursts of emotion ('emotionality' or 'emotional incontinence'). Performance on psychological testing is more patchy and more variable than for

Table 5.2 Ischaemic score – the Hachinski Scale

Feature	*Score*
Abrupt onset	2
Stepwise deterioration	1
Fluctuating course	2
Nocturnal confusion	1
Relative preservation of personality	1
Depression	1
Somatic complaints	1
Emotional incontinence (loss of emotional control)	1
History of hypertension	1
History of strokes	2
Evidence of associated atherosclerosis	1
Focal neurological symptoms	2
Focal neurological signs	2

Patients scoring 7 and above may be classified as having multi-infarct dementia, and patients scoring 4 and below may be classified as having primary degenerative dementia (probable AD).

AD with a particular tendency to increased confusion at night. Some of these characteristic features have been summed up by Hachinski in his scoring system (Table 5.2) which helps differentiate between AD and MID and has been confirmed by regional cerebral blood flow [12] and refined by pathological studies [13].

Not all psychological changes associated with stroke are harbingers of dementia and a patient with fluent dysphasia or marked emotionality who is otherwise well-preserved may become frustrated if labelled or treated as though demented.

(b) *Aetiology and pathology*

MID and acute onset vascular dementia are closely related to stroke illness and are associated with hypertension and atheroma. Most of the lesions are due to emboli (small blood clots) from the main arteries in the body. Hopefully, measures to reduce the prevalence of hypertension in the population will also reduce the incidence of MID, and treatments effective in reducing the incidence of recurrent stroke (e.g. low-dose aspirin) will slow the progression of MID. On pathological examination, the brains of sufferers contain multiple small or sometimes large areas of cerebral softening (infarcts) due to blocked blood vessels. There appears to be a 'threshold effect' with more than 50 ml of softening being associated with clinical dementia. In subcortical vascular dementia there are very small infarcts in the more central areas of brain tissue.

(c) Diagnosis

Again, this is largely from the history and mental state examination. Physical examination may reveal focal neurological changes, hypertension or other signs of vascular insufficiency. A CAT scan can help confirm the diagnosis; it will usually reveal areas of attenuation marking old infarctions. It may also show unsuspected subcortical infarcts in a patient with an apparent AD.

5.2.4 Other causes of dementia (mostly dealt with in ICD10; F02.8)

Although other causes of dementia are individually rare, they are important because some cases represent a subacute and potentially reversible confusional state rather than an irreversible dementia. The following list is not complete and the reader is referred to more comprehensive texts [14, 15] for a fuller account.

(a) Drugs

The tendency to issue a repeat prescription rather than examine the patient can cause great harm to old people. Many drugs, especially the benzodiazepines and drugs with anti-cholinergic effects, can cause confusion severe enough to precipitate a move from independent living to institutional care.

(b) Vitamin B12 deficiency

This is usually, but not always, associated with a megaloblastic anaemia. The patient's mental state may be indistinguishable from AD but an admixture of apparently depressive symptoms with marked slowing and apathy can sometimes give a clue.

Patients with AD may have lower than normal B12 levels and this may be one reason why the response to B12 injections is sometimes, though not always, disappointing. When there is a response, it is sometimes slow and incomplete (see Case history 5.1).

(c) Folic acid deficiency

Low serum folate levels are often an incidental finding in demented patients and are only rarely of aetiological significance. Red cell folate level is a better indicator of deficiency, being less affected by short-term dietary intake. Treatment with folic acid, which is cheap and may produce some benefit, is justified until diet can be improved.

(d) Thyroid deficiency

Coarsening of the hair, a puffy facial appearance, pre-tibial myxoedema and a deep voice may be noted but are not always present. The changes of hypothyroidism are sometimes so insidious that they are mistaken for normal ageing and when mental changes supervene, they are attributed to AD. Marked slowing and apathy are again characteristic, but treatment with gradually increasing doses of thyroxine often partially or fully restores mental function.

(e) Subdural haematoma

Chronic subdural haematoma is notoriously difficult to diagnose before death. The clinical picture may be of dementia or **delirium**. A high index of suspicion is essential and if there is a history of head injury or if the level of consciousness is varying markedly, an expert opinion and a CAT scan is justified.

(f) Other space-occupying lesions

Unexplained mental symptoms are sometimes due to intracranial growths. If these are malignant, they are often aggressive and declare themselves quickly. They are also often inoperable. Slow-growing, benign meningiomas can often mimic mental illness and a parasaggital meningioma can produce a picture quite similar to that of normal-pressure hydrocephalus.

(g) Normal-pressure hydrocephalus

This is characterized by the triad of confusion, abnormal gait and incontinence, more severe than would be expected in an early dementia. Patients presenting with this triad should be referred early for specialist assessment as an operation can sometimes reverse the disability.

(h) Alcoholic dementia (ICD10; F10.73)

The greatest risk factor among heavy drinkers for developing alcoholic dementia is increasing age. Disinhibition and impaired judgement are more common early in this form of dementia than in AD. Its progress may be arrested by abstention from alcohol. It may also be an accelerating factor in the deterioration due to MID or AD and may act as a risk factor for MID through the mechanism of hypertension. A history of excessive alcohol intake may be hard to elicit but hard-drinking friends or relatives, unexplained macrocytic anaemia or abnormal liver-function tests may provide a clue.

(i) Neurosyphilis

This is now a very rare cause of dementia in old age, but should not be discounted, especially if there is a relevant past history, or if the clinical picture is atypical. Serological tests can confirm or exclude the diagnosis.

(j) Dementia in human immunodeficiency virus (HIV) disease (ICD10; F02.4, also known as AIDS-dementia complex)

This condition is rare but not unheard of in old people. It presents with complaints of forgetfulness, slowness, and poor concentration or sometimes atypically with affective or psychotic symptoms. Progress of the disease is usually relatively quick (over weeks or months) to global dementia, mutism and death.

(k) Lewy-body dementia

Lewy bodies are microscopic pathological inclusions in brain tissue originally found in Parkinson's disease but now associated with a proportion of cases of apparent AD. There is still debate over how far a distinct clinical syndrome can be identified but Parkinsonian symptoms such as tremor, rigidity and slowed movement or prominent hallucinations may be markers. There appears to be a profound cholinergic deficit in Lewy-body dementia and it has been suggested that this form of dementia may be particularly likely to respond to treatment strategies based on enhancement of cholinergic neurotransmitters [16].

(l) Depressive pseudo-dementia

This is not really a true diagnostic term but serves as a useful reminder that some severely depressed patients, especially those with profound psychomotor retardation or agitation, may appear to be demented and may perform badly on memory tests. A history of relatively rapid onset, with loss of interest rather than loss of memory as the first symptom, and a positive personal or family history of affective illness are useful pointers. Patients with severe cognitive impairment during a depressive episode are more likely to develop dementia in the succeeding years, even though they make a good recovery with treatment of the initial episode.

(m) 'Cortical' and 'subcortical' dementia

A clinical distinction has been made between cortical and subcortical dementia. Alzheimer's dementia is the classic cortical dementia with marked aphasia, amnesia and impaired judgement. The subcortical dementias include the toxic and metabolic dementias and are characterized by forgetfulness, marked psychomotor slowing, apathetic or depressed mood, and often by abnormal posture, muscle tone and movements. Multi-infarct dementia often produces a mixed picture. The terms cortical and subcortical are anatomically misleading owing to the complicated interactions of systems within the brain. Nevertheless, they are clinically relevant, especially as so-called subcortical features can be an important clinical clue to an early and potentially treatable dementia.

> Case history 5.1:
>
> Mrs J.W. was an 83-year-old married woman who lived with her husband. About six years before presentation she had been admitted to a psychiatric ward with apparent depression. On this occasion, she was seen at home where she was in bed, almost stuporous, and apparently confused. Her husband said that she had been more or less normal until six weeks previously when she had started to deteriorate. A presumptive diagnosis of depressive pseudo-dementia was made but on admission she was found to have a profound megaloblastic anaemia with a B12 deficiency. Her mental state gradually improved with B12 injections but her memory was still far from perfect. However, when visited at home, she was able to find the drawer where the vials of neo-cytamen (B12) were kept.

Not all confusion is due to dementia, and not all mental slowing is due to depression. Figure 5.2 is a flow chart for the diagnosis of some of the most important causes of confusion.

5.3 MANAGEMENT

Specific psychological and pharmacological approaches will be discussed in Chapters 8 and 9. This section discusses the general approach to the problem of confusion. It is vital that the helper tries to understand how the patient experiences the problem. Patients, however confused, will have some residual abilities. In their attempts to make sense of their experience, they may cling to some inappropriate idea, for example, that they have to go home to make tea for the children. In delirium the patient may also feel frightened and threatened by attempts to help. The confused patient may easily be made anxious by changes in the environment and, in an attempt at self-preservation, may adopt a restricted lifestyle that resists intervention by would-be helpers.

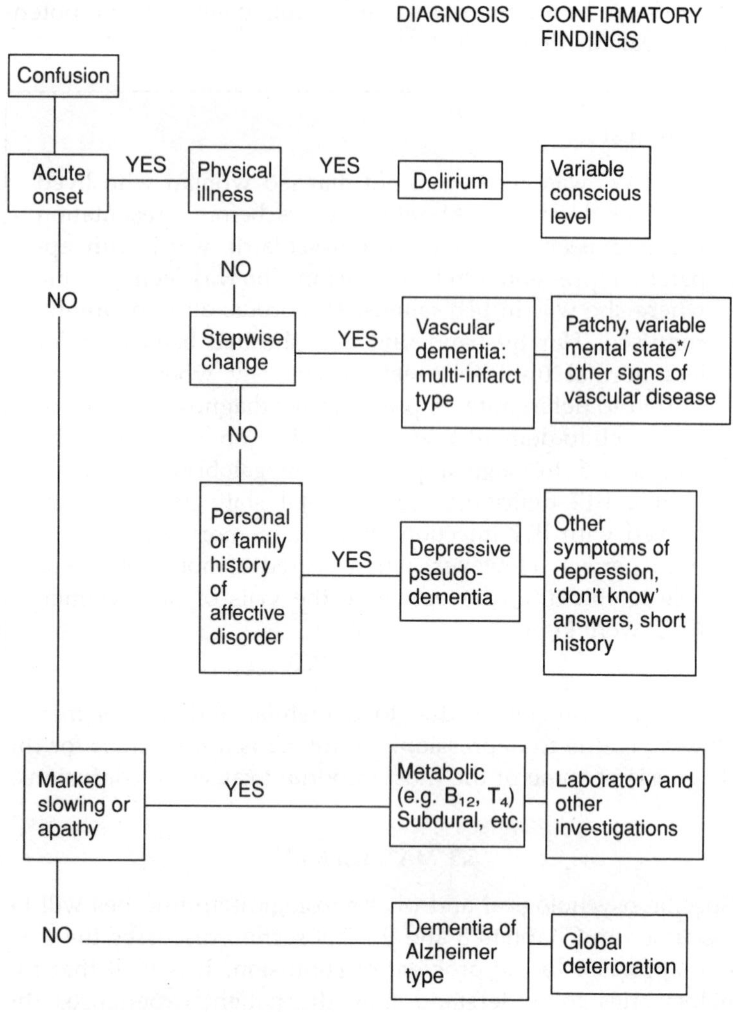

*Diffuse Lewy–Body disease also produces marked variability, often with visual hallucinations and/or extra-pyramidal symptoms

Figure 5.2 Flow chart for diagnosis of some important causes of confusion.

5.3.1 Analysing the problem

Figure 5.3 presents an interactive model of confusion which stresses that factors in the brain, the internal environment, the special senses and the external environment may all interact to cause confusion. In any one patient the contribution of environmental and personal factors will be unique and even where there is irreversible brain damage, treating the sufferer as a human being as well as attention to such factors as constipation, a malfunctioning hearing-aid and environmental design, may produce marked improvement. Brain-intrinsic factors and factors in the internal environment have already been discussed; special senses, the external environment and some specific points in management will be considered in the remainder of this chapter.

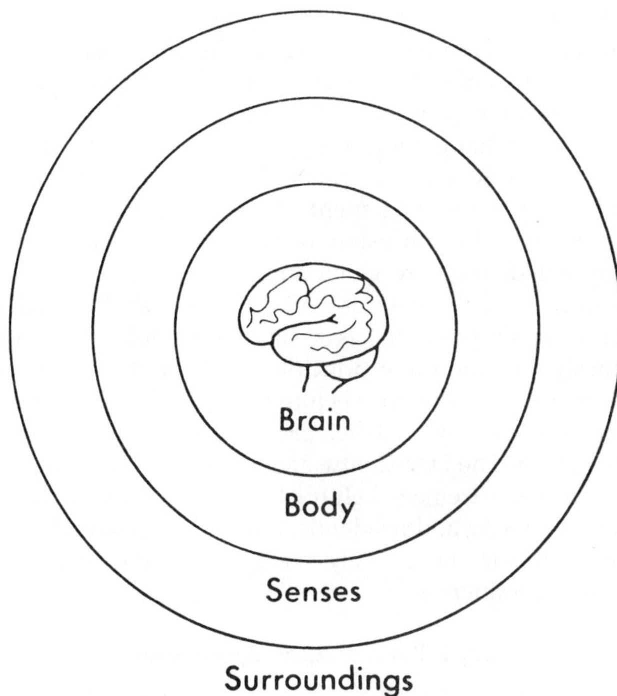

Figure 5.3 An interactive model of confusion.

5.3.2 Special senses

Sensory deprivation and distortion is used in 'brain-washing' and interrogation techniques to produce confusion and disorientation. Those of us who are blessed with good sight and hearing forget how confusing and frightening the world can be for an old person with poor hearing or sight. Disabilities in the special senses can combine with defects in other systems to render the old person extremely vulnerable. Imagine trying to cross a busy road with misty glasses, ear plugs and your ankles hobbled and you will get some idea of the predicament some old people find themselves in.

5.3.3 The external environment

A change of environment can provoke or worsen confusion, especially if badly managed. If an old person who is confused has to be subjected to a change of environment, for example an acute hospital admission or entering residential care, it is vital that the change is carefully managed. The old person should be prepared in advance. A familiar person should accompany her. As the transition proceeds, the person should be reminded about what is happening and where she is. Unfortunately, many old people enter residential care or hospital in crisis without adequate management of the change and an unnecessary increase in confusion occurs. When someone has a leg amputated, they are given an artificial leg or 'prosthesis'. In memory loss, the external environment can be used prosthetically. A shopping-list is a simple example of a memory 'prosthesis' but the same principle lies behind labels such as, 'Remember to lock the door before you go to bed,' 'Only cook a meal for one person,' and telephone calls, 'Hello, Mum – it's time to get up. The Day-Centre ambulance will be calling soon,' which can be extremely helpful to the person with mild dementia. In nursing and residential facilities, design and labelling can make toilets more easily recognizable and accessible so reducing incontinence.

5.3.4 Psychological approaches

Specific psychological approaches designed for the confused patient include reality orientation and validation therapy. Both of these approaches depend on recognizing the cognitive and emotional impact of dementia on the individual and trying to alleviate this. They are discussed further in Chapter 8.

5.3.5 The personal touch

Every confused person faces a unique set of problems and has a unique set of experiences to help in coping with them. The logical analysis of problems is one side of the coin and treating the person with dementia as a valued individual the other. Systematic analysis and treatment of incidental problems like constipation, poor hearing and the lack of a regular routine including appropriate social support helps. Above all, treating the sufferer as a person not a problem works wonders. Relatives also deserve special consideration. In addition to the strains imposed by problems of wandering, incontinence or unpredictable behaviour, they face the emotional stress of 'living bereavement' and may be worn down by the need for 24-hour care, 365 days a year. They need practical help such as arranging attendance allowance or day care but often they also need emotional support such as can be provided by a relatives' support group run by professionals or by a voluntary body such as the Alzheimer's Disease Society.

5.3.6 Drugs

There is no drug yet discovered which has been shown to arrest the progress of AD or MID or reliably produce clinically significant improvement in the mental state of patients suffering from these diseases. The discovery that the cholinergic neurotransmitter systems are particularly affected in AD led to a search for a 'replacement therapy' analagous to the use of L-dopa in Parkinson's disease. Choline and its precursor lecithin have been given to demented patients but the results have been generally disappointing. Anti-cholinesterase drugs and cholinergic agonists have also been tried without any major success as yet. Other neurotransmitter-enhancing drugs are in development and mono-amine oxidase-B inhibitors and nerve growth factor are being evaluated for possible neuro-protective effects. At present, however, there is no specific treatment. Symptomatic treatment with drugs should be avoided when-

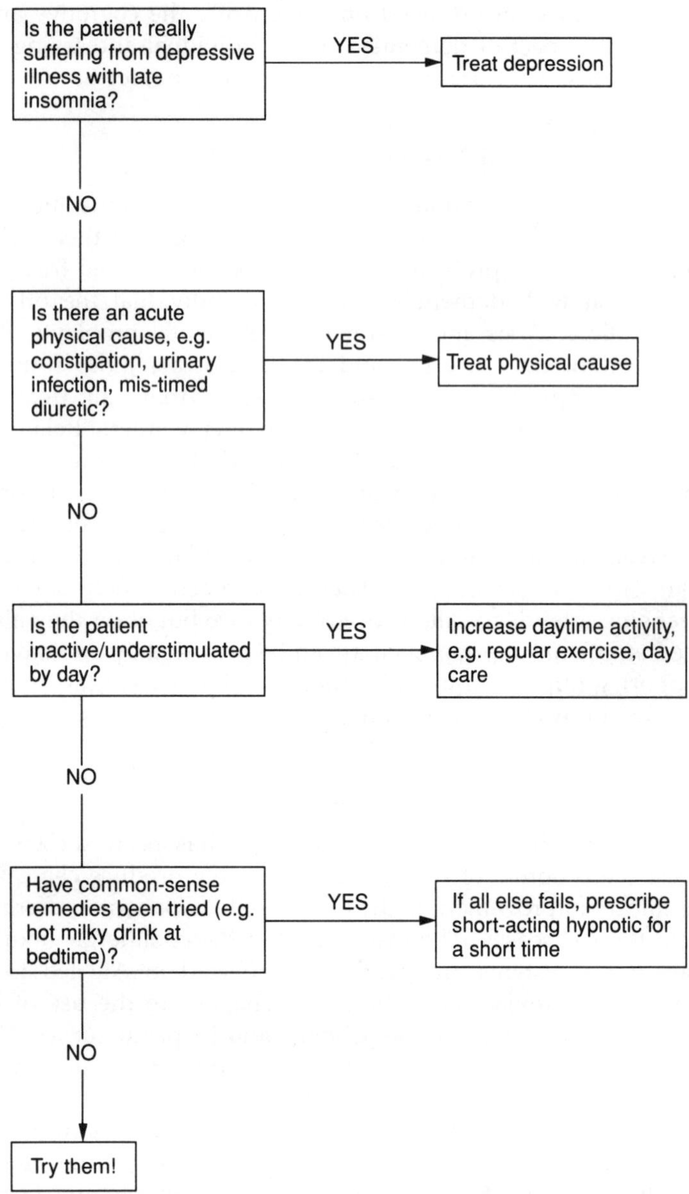

Figure 5.4 Management of insomnia in an elderly confused patient.

ever possible because of the risk of adverse effects, though anti-depressants and neuroleptics may be indicated sometimes (see Chapter 9).

5.3.7 Specific problems

Sleep disturbance, wandering, unco-operativeness, aggression, shouting, dangerous behaviour and other specific problems occur in the context of dementia. If an elderly confused patient is sleepless at night, this can be the last straw for caring relatives. Nevertheless, other approaches should be tried before drugs. This is illustrated in Figure 5.4.

Wandering is a common problem. Some demented patients wander in a fairly reliable and safe way around their places of residence and should be allowed to do so. Others are a danger to themselves and other people and the wandering has to be controlled. We had a patient who was discovered more than once wandering on the M1 – it had not been there when she was younger! If common-sense measures (e.g. more directed exercise, other occupation, or treating constipation) fail, then more sophisticated behavioural management may be needed (see Chapter 8). Drugs are a last resort. Their use is discussed in Chapter 9. People who are causing danger by driving while significantly impaired need to be persuaded to give up their licences or, if necessary, to be reported to the licensing authorities.

5.3.8 Other measures

Relatives of demented patients often complain that the disease has not been explained to them and that they do not know what to expect. When making an initial assessment of a confused patient, the needs of the relatives or caregivers for information and support should be considered. In some areas, organizations like the Alzheimer's Disease Society run local telephone help-lines and national help-lines are also available but these should be regarded as a supplement rather than an alternative to the individual assessment and advice of the clinician.

Relatives who are going through a period of 'living bereavement' may need appropriate counselling. This is a role that various professionals may be trained to take. At other times, illness in old age will expose stresses that have been present in a marriage for many years. Sometimes, but by no means always, this may be amenable to a counselling or psychotherapeutic approach.

Different members of the primary care team and of the specialist multi-disciplinary team (MDT) for old age psychiatry, such as doctors, community psychiatric nurses, social workers, psychologists and occupational therapists all have special skills to offer. Practical services such as day care, home care, ready-made meals, laundry and incontinence services, respite care, family care and other help can enhance the coping ability of the patient and her relatives. With so many different professionals, voluntary and other care agencies and relatives potentially involved, good communication is vital. In the UK, the Community Care Act and the new contracting process for fundholding general practices, stress the need for service providers to prepare individual care-programmes for patients.

While this is good advice, some of the procedures developed to enable this to happen **and to be centrally monitored** are very labour intensive and impossible to achieve within existing resources. Though case-conferences may be ideal for gathering and sharing information and developing a management programme, telephone liaison may be more practicable with limited resources. Sadly, statutory community services are very variable. Whereas in some places the home-help service or the district nurse may be able to attend daily to ensure the patient is ready for the Day Centre or to administer medication to someone living alone, in other areas none of these services will be available. The availability and quality of hospital-based services remains variable, despite the rapid development of specialist services in recent years.

5.4 CONCLUSION

In this chapter we have adopted an interactive model for understanding the needs of confused old people. We have considered the way in which physical, psychological and environmental factors interact to generate or worsen confusion. We have stressed that, even when confusion is due to an irreversible dementia, there may well be interventions that can be made to improve the patient's function and the quality of life of patient and caregivers. We would argue that good health and social care for confused old people is a measure of the quality of our civilization and, sadly, at present is a measure which finds us wanting.

REFERENCES

1. Hofman, A., Rocca, W.A. and Amaducci, L. (1991) A collaborative study of the prevalence of dementia in Europe: the Eurodem findings, in *Diagnostic and Therapeutic Assessment in Alzheimer's Disease*, (eds C.G. Gottfries, R. Levy, G. Clincke and L. Tritsams), Wrightson Biomedical Publishing, Petersfield.
2. Blessed, G. and Wilson, I.D. (1982) The contemporary natural history of mental disorder in old age. *British Journal of Psychiatry*, **141**, 59–67.
3. Dick, D.H. (1982) *The Rising Tide: Developing Services for Mental Illness in Old Age*, National Health Service, Health Advisory Service, Sutton.
4. *Care of Elderly People with Mental Illness: Specialist Services and Medical Training* (1989) The Royal College of Physicians of London and the Royal College of Psychiatrists, London.
5. Gilleard, C.J. (1992) Carers: recent research findings, in *Recent Advances in Psychogeriatrics* (2) (ed. T. Arie), Churchill Livingstone, Edinburgh, pp 137–52.
6. Kitwood, T. and Bredin, K. (1992) Towards a theory of dementia care: personhood and well being. *Ageing and Society*, **12**, 269–87.
7. Kitwood, T. and Bredin, K. (1992) *Person to Person: a Guide to the Care of those with Failing Mental Powers*, Gale Centre Publications, Loughton.
8. Kitwood, T. and Bredin, K. (1992) A new approach to the evaluation of dementia care. *Journal of Advances in Health and Nursing Care*, **1** (5), 41–60.
9. Christie, A. and Wood, E. (1990) Further changes in the pattern of mental disorders in the elderly. *British Journal of Psychiatry*, **157**, 228–31.
10. Blessed, G., Tomlinson, B.E. and Roth, M. (1968) The association between quantitative measures of dementia and senile change in the grey matter of elderly people. *British Journal of Psychiatry*, **144**, 797–811.
11. Rossor, M.N., Iversen, L.L., Reynolds, G.P. *et al*. (1984) Neurochemical characteristics of early and late onset types of Alzheimer's disease. *British Medical Journal*, **288**, 961–4.
12. Hachinski, V.C., Illiff, L.D., Zilka, E. *et al*. (1975) Cerebral blood flow in dementia. *Archives of Neurology*, **32**, 632–7.
13. Rosen, W.G., Terry, R.D., Fuld, P.A. *et al*. (1980) Pathological verification of ishaemic score in differentiation of dementias. *Annals of Neurology*, **5**, 486–8.

14. Lishman, W.A. (1987) *Organic Psychiatry: the Psychological Consequences of Cerebral Disorder*, Blackwell Scientific Publications, Oxford.
15. Cummings, J.L. and Benson, D.F. (1983) *Dementia, a Clinical Approach*, Butterworth, Boston.
16. Byrne, E.J. (1992) Diffuse Lewy–Body disease, spectrum disorder or variety of Alzheimer's disease? *International Journal of Geriatric Psychiatry*, **7**, 229–34.

6

Somatization and hypochondriasis

Nearly everyone who is reading this sentence will, after a moment's thought, be able to isolate some area of mild discomfort or pain in their own body. Indeed, it is estimated that some three out of four people have symptoms in any given month which lead them to take action such as medicating themselves, resting in bed or visiting their GPs. The pattern we expect is that a symptom leads to an appropriate course of action. An appropriate response is defined by what we know of the symptom type, severity and a number of other factors, such as the type of activity the person would do if not ill. For example, athletes in training, pregnant women or staff working with children or sick people might be expected to behave in certain ways other people might not consider, to maintain fitness or protect others. Levels of complaints, avoidance of activity, requests for care and compliance with treatment are all taken into account by each of us as part of the normal monitoring of events in ourselves and those around us. Many of us do not usually let the presence of mild pain or discomfort interfere with our leisure activities or work: we communicate about our symptoms and accept care and reassurance from friends, relatives or a doctor. To this extent, illness behaviour is ubiquitous and normal. Some individuals do not fit our expectations of normal illness behaviour.

Old people probably somatize more than young ones: that is, they complain of a physical symptom rather than emotional distress. Old people are also more likely to be assumed to be hypochondriacal. This may be generational, in that they have been less exposed to psychology. In any case, old people are certainly more likely to be suffering from a number of physical symptoms than young people. There is therefore a need when working within psychiatric services for old people to be familiar with the range of ways in which a complaint about a physical symptom can be understood and treated. In this chapter, the authors will discuss not only the range of conditions but will focus also on psychological models which have been used to explain or treat people suffering from fears of illness and other complaints.

The ICD10 [1] classification outlines a number of disorders in which beliefs about physical symptoms or illness are features. These include depression (F33.0.01, F33.1.01), considered in Chapter 4, and the somatoform disorders (F45), which include somatization disorder (F45.0), undifferentiated somatoform disorder (F45.1), hypochondriasis (F45.2), somatoform autonomic dysfunction (F45.3), persistent somatoform pain disorder (F45.4) and others (F45.8). The existence of these terms and the range of competing diagnoses highlight the complexity of the relationship between the body, the mind and behaviour.

6.1 THE SOMATOFORM DISORDERS (F45)

The core feature of the group of somatoform disorders is repetitious presentation of physical symptoms, along with requests for medical investigations, in the face of repeated negative findings and reassurances by doctors that the symptoms have no physical basis. When there is physical illness, it is considered insufficient to explain the severity of distress and the extent of concern of the patient. Even if there are clear precipitating life events, the patient does not countenance a link between these and the presentation of physical complaints, even when there are clear symptoms of anxiety or depression. Difficulties in coming to a mutually acceptable understanding of the symptoms can lead to frustration for both doctor and patient. Histrionic behaviour is often a feature when the patient becomes resentful at their failure to persuade doctors that their illness has a physical basis and requires more investigation.

6.1.1 Somatization disorder (F45.0)

The main features are multiple, recurrent and changing symptoms, usually present for several years before referral into a psychiatric service (over two years for a diagnosis). There may be a long history of fruitless investigations and treatments, resulting in a 'fat file'. Reassurance from several doctors has to be unsuccessful for this diagnosis to be made. Symptoms may be attributed to all body parts, but perhaps gastro-intestinal and skin complaints are among the most common. Somatization is associated with the disruption of social, interpersonal and family behaviour. Anxiety, depression and secondary dependence on medication may be present and may have to be treated separately. Undifferentiated somatoform disorder (F45.1) is a less clearly defined category in which some of the characteristics of the above are absent.

6.1.2 Hypochondriacal disorders (F45.2)

Hypochondriasis is defined as a persistent preoccupation with the possibility of serious, progressive disease. Patients complain of physical symptoms or of their appearance. Commonplace or normal sensations are interpreted as distressing or abnormal, and there may be a focus on a particular area. The patient may name the disease they fear. Anxiety and depression are commonly present and the course of the complaints is chronic but fluctuates. Referral to psychiatry is often resented and associated disability is variable. The reassurance of several doctors has no effect. This diagnostic category excludes delusional disorders.

These are distinguished from somatization disorders by clarifying the focus of the patient's concern; a somatizing patient will ask for removal of the symptoms and comply well with drug treatment at least for periods, a hypochondriacal one will be concerned with the underlying disease from which they feel they are suffering, and may mistrust medication in spite of continued requests for investigation. Anxiety and panic disorders may have a similar presentation.

The somatoform disorders also include the following categories, from which old people are not immune:

6.1.3 Somatoform autonomic dysfunction (F45.3)

The patient presents symptoms as if they are due to a physical disorder of a system or organ under autonomic control, i.e. cardiovascular, gastro-intestinal or respiratory system disease.

Common types in old people are cardiac neurosis, psychogenic hyperventilation and bowel dysfunction. Two types of symptom are offered: those attributable to autonomic arousal, such as sweating, palpitations and tremor, and those which are more idiosyncratic, subjective or non-specific. These are referred to a particular organ. There may also be signs of stress or current problems. Again, repeated reassurance by doctors is unsuccessful; no underlying physical disease is found.

6.1.4 Persistent somatoform pain disorder (F45.4)

This means that the patient complains of persistent, severe and distressing pain, to a degree inexplicable by a physical or physiological process. There are links with present psycho-social problems or emotional conflict and there is an increase in support or attention.

6.1.5 Other somatoform disorders (F45.8, F45.9)

These categories include symptoms such as disorders of skin sensation, globus hystericus, and psychogenic pruritus, limited to a specific system and unrelated to tissue damage (F45.8), and other unspecified disorders (F45.9).

Other diagnostic categories relevant to the chapter include:

6.1.6 Neurasthenia (F48.0)

This category includes two major variations, fatigue after either mental or physical effort. There are often accompanying reports of dizziness, tension headaches and a sense of general instability, while concern about lowering health, irritability, anhedonia and low-level depression or anxiety are common. There may be changes in the duration (hypersomnia) or pattern (disturbance in the early and middle stages) of sleep.

6.1.7 Psychological and behavioural factors associated with disorders or disease classified elsewhere (F54)

This category concerns the presence of psychological or behavioural influences thought to have played a significant part in the aetiology of a physical condition. In cases defined as within this category, resulting mental disturbances are minor and do not rate a diagnostic category in themselves. The physical illnesses commonly associated with this category include asthma, eczema and dermatitis, gastric ulcer, colitis and urticaria.

6.2 FACTORS AFFECTING ASSESSMENT OF THE SOMATOFORM DISORDERS IN OLD PEOPLE

6.2.1 Physical illness

Clinical studies suggest that hypochondriasis should not be viewed as a unitary syndrome, but as a phenomenon which is frequently associated with a treatable psychiatric or medical state [2]. The first step in the effective management of elderly people with hypochondriacal complaints or other somatoform disorder is the identification and treatment of such illnesses.

Sometimes a diagnosis of hypochondriasis or hysteria is made, but on examination of the patient there are clear signs of physical illness that was originally missed because of the way in which the patient presented. The importance of the context in which a complaint is made cannot be overestimated. The assumptions of relatives and the health professionals are based on complex belief systems which include ideas about what health in old age is like, and what behaviour is appropriate for a patient or sick family member.

One difficulty common to many old people is the presence of one or more chronic illnesses. It is sometimes difficult to determine whether the existing disease may explain new symptoms. Some of the most common illnesses of old age, including vascular and joint changes for example, are not curable. These may have profound secondary effects on general levels of fitness and other conditions. Some patients may suffer from both physical disease and psychiatric pathology [3].

In addition, they are likely to suffer from a larger number of symptoms related to major or minor illnesses. These need to be carefully distinguished from complaints that have no basis in physical illness. The joke in which a patient replies to the doctor's reassurance that it is, 'Just your age' with, 'Well, my other leg is 90 as well and that's causing me no problem,' comes to mind. One difficulty when treating the hypochondriacal patient lies in the difficulty of dealing with their demands without becoming frustrated. This can at worst lead to brusque or punitive treatment, or to refusals to investigate complaints and occasional missed diagnoses. Hypochondriacs can get ill, too!

Physical examination should be thorough and appear to be thorough to the patient. Saying in a gentle tone of voice, 'I can understand that you feel you are ill but there is really not anything seriously wrong with you', is better than entering into an argument with the patient which will only raise her anxiety level still further and exacerbate her physical symptoms. Many patients suspect that their doctors are not telling them everything: hardly surprising, perhaps, as some doctors do have a policy not to inform patients of a fatal diagnosis, despite the fact that studies indicate most people would rather have such information than not.

Once a patient is labelled as hypochondriacal there is a danger that because she has had one complete examination recently the doctor assumes that subsequent complaints are hypochondriacal in nature: the patient cries wolf once too often! In one case a 67-year-old woman living with her brother was diagnosed as having pneumonia by one of the authors during a psychiatric domiciliary visit requested by the GP. Her hypochondriasis pre-dated the pneumonia. After the pneumonia responded to treatment, she still remained difficult to manage and was diagnosed as suffering from a depressive illness. She remained non-compliant to treatment for months but was eventually admitted to hospital and agreed to a course of ECT, to which her depression responded. Before assigning this type of psychiatric diagnosis to an old person, therefore, caution is advisable.

There is some evidence that physical examination on request (within reason), when carried out promptly and thoroughly in response to acute hypochondriacal fears, reduces anxiety, although the relief does not persist for long. In practice, it may reinforce the behaviour of requesting physical examinations.

6.2.2 Affective disorder

After a full physical investigation and with continued monitoring of physical state, the next step is to ascertain whether or not the hypochondriasis is part of an affective disorder. There is a clear and strong association between hypochondriasis and affective disorder. De Alaracon found that nearly two-thirds of 152 consecutive depressed patients admitted to a geriatric unit had hypochondriacal symptoms [4]. The importance of identifying the elderly person who presents with hypochondriasis as part of a depressive illness cannot be over-stressed, not just because there are effective treatments for depression, but because of the high risk of suicide attempts (over a third in De Alaracon's study) in depressed elderly people who show hypochondriasis as the dominant symptom.

Digestive symptoms, ranging from intense over-concern about constipation to delusions about the cessation of bowel movement and about head and facial pain, are by far the most frequent hypochondriacal symptoms associated with depression in the aged [4, 5]. Other preoccupations may concern cardiovascular, urinary and genital areas of the body. Complaints about skin and hair, for example that handfuls of hair are falling out, seem to be largely confined to women. From the authors' own experience, identification of a depressive illness masquerading as a hypochondriasis is difficult in some cases. The doctor needs to assess, through direct questioning, the patient's mood and mental state, looking for the presence of sleep disturbance, depressive thoughts, suicidal ideas and loss of energy and interest in life, family, work and hobbies. The recent, rapid onset of hypochondriacal symptoms in a person who has never previously had such symptoms, should be regarded as a possible indicator of affective disorder. Where an elderly person has shown life-long hypochondriacal behaviour with a fondness for unnecessary medication, etc., a depressive episode may be signalled by a dramatic change in intensity of concern or in the nature and content of worries. Of all patients, those who have hypochondriacal complaints concerning facial or head pain are perhaps the most likely to show an atypical presentation of a depressive illness [6].

6.2.3 Health complaints and hypochondriasis in old people

While hypochondriasis is defined as a severe anxiety about one's health, expressed as a fear of having or a belief that one has, a physical illness, other people may have health anxieties to a lesser extent. Many, perhaps even the majority of medical consultations are made by patients for whom the symptom alone does not fully explain the distress [7]. This may not seem surprising; even minor illness may significantly disrupt a daily routine and cause a number of 'hassles' at just the time when they are hardest to deal with. Old people often live with health anxieties of varying types and duration. Elderly people who are hypochondriacal sometimes show a degree and type of distressed behaviour which is not only difficult for friends and relatives, but also presents apparently insurmountable problems to the doctor and other professionals. There seem to be a number of related factors arising during the process of ageing which might account for this.

As individuals age there will be an increasing build-up of minor physical lesions which can become the focus of the hypochondriacal complaint. Not only this, they will have more direct experience of those close to them suffering serious or terminal illnesses. Such experiences can heighten anxiety both directly, by raising fears of death or of helplessness, and indirectly, by increasing isolation from meaningful relationships and activities. Where the general level of anxiety is raised there is a danger that minor aches and pains can be perceived as more extreme or as serious illness. It is not unusual to find a minor physical lesion at the site of the hypochondriacal complaint, or that the nature of the complaint is of the same kind as the terminal illness which a close relative suffered.

6.3 PSYCHIATRIC MANAGEMENT OF THE SOMATIZING PATIENT

6.3.1 Physical treatments

A number of approaches exist for the treatment of patients with health anxieties. In addition to the physical treatments for depression and anxiety, a number of drugs are thought to have specific effects on such symptomatology, e.g. pimozide for the patient who expresses a specific delusional anxiety about disease. When an anti-depressant is indicated, the newer 'SSRI' drugs (see Chapter 9) may be preferred because they produce relatively fewer side-effects.

For some patients, the acceptability and success of treatment can be affected by bearing in mind simple psychological principles. A clear formulation may help other professionals involved with the case, as well as the patient. Other patients may benefit from either an individual psychological approach or from work carried out with their family. This is discussed further on in the chapter.

Changes in medication can have a significant effect. Paradoxically, it seems that the reduction or removal of some long-standing prescriptions can have beneficial effects. Notable in this respect are sleeping medications and hypnotics, which can adversely affect the quality and duration of sleep, and laxatives, which can affect bowel function and lead to abdominal pain. The effect of giving such medications over a period is not limited to side-effects. Without education about the rationale for a sleeping tablet, for example, the patient may believe that a full night's sleep is an essential requirement for health and may continue to be intolerant of reductions even over a short period, leading to worries about the problem, to demands for an increase or change of prescription or to other strategies which lead to further problems, such as catnapping to make up for 'lost' sleep. Giving medication may in itself lead the patient to worry that there is an underlying serious disease; after all, something has to warrant tablets.

Catnapping is one example of a range of lifestyle factors which may affect bodily functioning. These include dietary intake; for example, fibre affects bowel function. Caffeine affects levels of arousal; this effect may increase with age (the authors certainly find this so!). Exercise has a number of beneficial effects, on general well-being and on bowel function and sleep. Alcohol, nicotine and other drugs can produce a number of adverse effects. It may be possible to alter some symptoms significantly through changing these. Insomnia is a common health complaint of old people. Table 6.1 outlines some of the possible strategies for helping someone deal with this problem [8].

Whenever there is a physical illness, the emphasis should be to explain any treatment clearly and simply. However, despite the best efforts of the physician, this may be a frustrating experience, as the patient may interpret the information given to support the possibility of disease, while even the mildest of side-effects arising from treatment may be magnified out of all proportion, because of the patients' hypersensitivity to changes

Table 6.1 Assessment and possible strategies for overcoming insomnia

1. Assessment to include:	
environmental changes	
medication	
sleep pattern	
anxieties	
beliefs about sleep	
2. Treatment may include:	
education about sleep	– how much is necessary what happens if sleep is reduced
changing behaviours that might impair sleep	– increase exercise – reducing stimulants such as tea or coffee at night – stopping catnaps – sticking to a routine
cognitive strategies	– identify worries about not sleeping and refute – taking steps towards the solution of other worries
relaxation strategies	– progressive relaxation
making bedtime conducive to sleep	– procedures, rituals, avoiding activities other than sleep in bed

in their own body state. Invasive tests are particularly risky in this respect, and the physician should be fully aware of the possible consequences of such testing.

6.3.2 Information, explanation and examination

Elderly people presenting in a state of anxiety in a medical setting are no different from younger people in that they may easily misinterpret or forget what is being said to them. Some beliefs about health within the population as a whole are erroneous or inaccurate. We have only to think about the prejudices which abound about HIV infection, for example. This can be illustrated by referring to one study on beliefs about peptic-ulcer formation, which found that while most patients had a clear idea that acid was important in ulcer formation, only ten per cent had realized that acid was secreted by the stomach, some thinking it came from the teeth when food was chewed and others from the brain when food was swallowed [9]. Older people may be less likely to seek out or take in such information about their health, as is common knowledge among young professionals. Information should be kept simple and if possible written down. It is important to avoid the use of technical terms. It is also likely that elderly patients will have minor discomforts with impressive labels, for example sinusitis or gastritis. These may be misunderstood as being the reason for their hypochondriacal complaints, and their possible implications should be simply explained and clarified.

One common area of misunderstanding by staff is the hypochondriacal patients' experience of pain. Thus patients may still be told they are 'imagining' the pain because there is no physical lesion or that the pain is psychological. In fact pain is a subjective experience and as such should be accepted as being real for the patient who reports it [10].

In summary, then, clarity and simplicity of information, and physical examinations at regular intervals, may help to reduce anxiety and may reduce the level of hypochondriacal complaints. Some psychotherapeutic approaches have emphasized these aspects of treatment [11]. Even when the hypochondriasis is part of a depressive illness, this approach is important because it facilitates the patient's trust and confidence which will improve compliance with any necessary treatment.

6.4 DEPRESSIVE HYPOCHONDRIASIS

Where a depressive illness may be present, any intervention, whether psychological or physical, should be based on a testable hypothesis about the nature and causes of the hypochondriasis, should be time limited, and should be used as an assessment of the nature of the disorder. For example, in a married couple, it is not always easy to assess the degree to which the hypochondriacal complaints arise from marital arguments through the exacerbation of anxiety, rather than from a depressive illness which then undermines a fragile marital harmony. As has been emphasized in other chapters the possibility of successful treatment can be maximized through the use of carefully planned and timed interventions considering all the relevant physical, psychiatric, psychological and

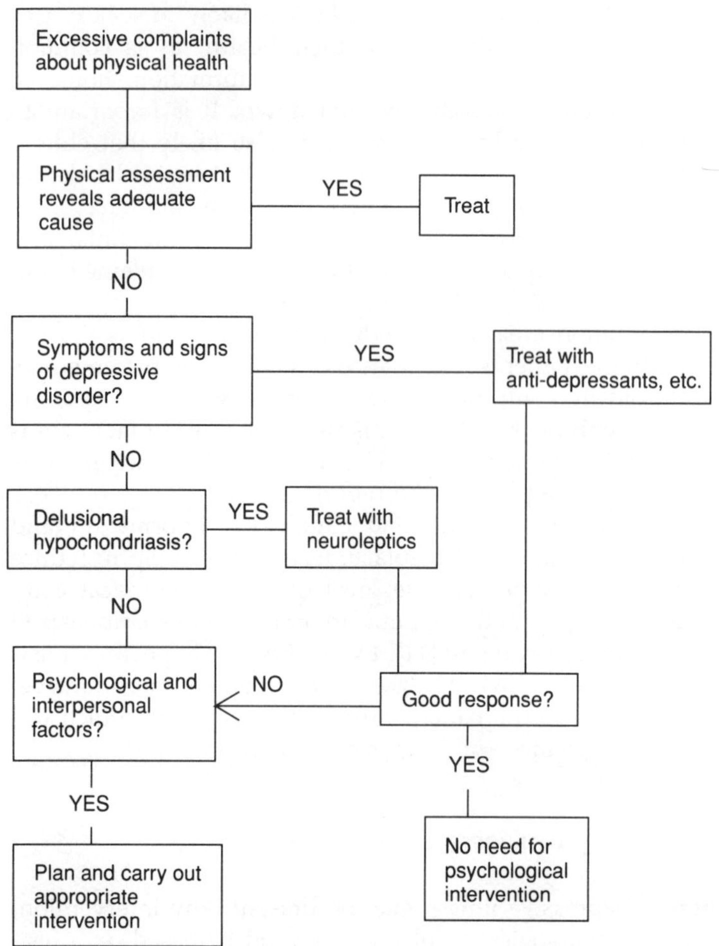

Figure 6.1 Simplified flow chart for deciding on treatment approach in a patient presenting with excessive health anxiety.

social factors. Figure 6.1 outlines a strategy for assessment of a patient with hypochondriacal complaints.

Many of those depressed patients with predominant hypochondriasis show particularly poor compliance with physical psychiatric treatments, perhaps because they believe they are not being treated appropriately. A clear and co-ordinated management plan is of paramount importance in these cases. At its core should be a consistent response by the psychiatric team to make the acceptance of necessary treatment for depression more, rather than less, likely. A pattern of repeated admission and discharge, during which the person never complies adequately with any treatment offered, should be resisted. Admission should normally only take place with the agreement of the patient to a clear contract to accept a particular treatment, not because, for example, the spouse cannot cope any longer with the partner's complaints. While coercion is generally undesirable, the alternative may be to leave the elderly person in distress for months at a time because the hypochondriacal behaviour prevents the implementation of effective physical treatment. Since the GP may receive the bulk of the hypochondriacal complaints, he must be fully involved in the psychiatric team's management plan.

The case history presented next illustrates how difficult the treatment of such a patient can be. A number of approaches were tried, none alone proving sufficient.

Case history 6.1:

Mrs F.V. was a 67-year-old married woman who was taken over by our team one month after being discharged from a psychiatric ward where incomplete treatment with anti-depressants, one application of ECT and attempts at marital therapy had failed. She had a three-year history of physical complaints, apparently precipitated by having her ears pierced, and previous physical investigations included a nose biopsy. Interestingly, her main presenting symptom was of pain in her nose but there was also ear and mouth pain, chest pain, swollen ankles, athlete's foot and worries about her diabetes for which she received a daily injection from a district nurse. It was 'catch 22' for the staff involved: on the one hand Mrs F.V. demanded help for her physical condition, yet every treatment attempt made, whether it was anti-depressant medication, pain killers or soothing ear drops, resulted in an apparent exacerbation of her symptoms, possibly because of hypersensitivity to small changes in her bodily state, and then non-compliance.

Mrs F.V.'s ambivalence towards medication led to initial attempts at a psychological intervention. Marital work was impossible because of Mrs F.V.'s preoccupation with her physical state which was occasionally interspersed with heated arguments with her husband; and individual work with Mr F.V. to try to reduce the level of his expressed anger and increase his coping skills failed because of his inability to comply. As he put it, he could cope much better at Dunkirk with his friends being killed around him than with his wife in this condition.

Two admissions ensued, both of which were characterized by lack of compliance. After her discharge from the second admission the team agreed to resist further admissions until she consented to a full course of ECT. There was a gradual and eventually very marked change in Mrs F.V. over eleven sessions of ECT. Her complaints diminished, although she still reported some ear and mouth pain, and her level of interest and activity greatly increased. After the sixth ECT, marital work was again instituted with the aim of preparing Mr and Mrs F.V. for a resumption in normal life, as Mr F.V. had taken over most of his wife's role as a housewife. Also, ways in which both could express their affection more directly to each other were explored, and nursing staff encouraged Mrs F.V. to be more independent regarding her physical health by teaching her to self-administer her insulin. Mr and Mrs F.V. did not wish to attend regularly for marital work after her discharge, but Mrs F.V. maintained her improvement at two-month follow-up. A year later she relapsed, following a physical illness, but readily agreed to come into hospital for a course of ECT and maintenance anti-depressants, to which she responded rapidly and completely.

Whenever possible the person should be encouraged to manage independently as far as is possible. In this case, the progression from dependence on a district nurse for her insulin injection to self-administration of her insulin and monitoring of her urine sugar level were important, both for Mrs F.V.'s self-esteem and the total amount of health services' input.

6.5 PSYCHOLOGICAL FACTORS

A person's beliefs influence behaviour and vice versa. Looking at this inter-relationship and its consequences on a person's emotional state is the basis of cognitive therapy, the use of which has been expanded into a number of areas, including that of the treatment of health anxiety and the psychological aspects of illness [12]. For treatment purposes, Salkovskis [13] defines three categories of somatic disorders: those people whose presentations include observable and identifiable disturbances of bodily functioning, e.g. irritable bowel, sleep disorder; those where the disturbance can be seen as perceptual, with sensitivity or excessive reaction to normal bodily sensation, e.g. hypochondriasis, somatization disorder; and a mixed group, to include headache, breathlessness, pain and cardiac neurosis.

When considering a psychological intervention, it is important to estimate the extent to which health anxiety is a major part of the problem. Beliefs about health may have an effect on the patient's understanding of the appropriate treatment and on compliance with treatment, so that the degree of success in dealing with anxieties about health may influence further interventions.

Salkovskis also lists the factors which maintain health anxieties. These are outlined in Table 6.2.

Table 6.2 Factors which maintain health anxieties

i) increased physiological arousal, which has effects such as palpitations, sweating or gastro-intestinal disturbance;
ii) the patient's focus of attention alters so that normal variations in bodily function are seen as new and symptomatic; this may lead to changes in physiological functioning;
iii) avoidant behaviours to minimize physical discomfort and to prevent dangerous illness, e.g. avoiding activity to prevent a heart attack;
iv) misinterpretations of symptoms, signs and medical communications in line with the patient's existing beliefs about their condition, which hinder the patient from accepting reassurance.

6.5.1 Psychological assessment

This is often made more difficult because the patient believes that there is a physical illness and does not welcome the thought of either a psychological or psychiatric assessment. The patient's ideas about the assessment itself are important. For example, a patient may believe that the referral has been made because they have been a nuisance with their complaints, or because the doctor thinks their complaint is fictitious. In this case, it may be helpful to explain that there are a number of physical illnesses for which psychological approaches can be helpful, by, for example, reducing stress and helping a person cope better with their illness. It is important at the start at least not to challenge the patient's views of their condition but to present with an open mind as to the nature of the problem and the appropriate treatment, offering the assessment as an assurance that all possible options are being explored.

It is important to let the patient talk about and explore with them their beliefs about their illness. This may allow important information to become apparent, such as antecedents to the symptoms, such as external events, thoughts or behaviours. When the symptoms are present or becoming worse, the patient is asked about their thoughts, including mental images and predictions, and their actions, including going home from work, going to bed, phoning someone for reassurance or help, watching television to distract themselves. Discussing beliefs about illness in general and about doctors can be useful. Some people also have strategies for protecting themselves by avoiding something, such as refusing to go out of the house in cold weather.

Patients can be asked to monitor or keep records of their symptoms, the preceding events or thoughts, and subsequent actions or events, along with their effects. This can provide valuable information about the nature of the problem, which can then be used in designing and implementing treatments. It also provides record of the degree of symptomatology, so that changes over time can be monitored.

Psychological interviews such as this differ from diagnostic interviews because they do not aim for a psychiatric diagnosis, but instead to come to a psychological formulation which includes the patient's beliefs, behaviours and the effects of these.

6.5.2 Psychological treatment

Treatment can only proceed if it is acceptable to the patient, so a great deal of skill has to be put into making a formulation of the problem and in defining treatment goals that satisfy both a psychologically minded therapist and an illness-minded patient. This may mean accepting the reality of the patient's experience, but asking them to try out something new for a limited period. If the approach does not help them after a time, then they are free to go back to their old strategies. In the initial contract, it is explained that the therapist will help them look for and test out alternatives reasons for their symptoms and that medical checks and lengthy discussions of the symptoms will not be part of the treatment.

Change is more likely to occur with any patient if there is a therapeutic relationship in which the patient feels that the professional respects her point of view. The patient will probably already have experience of reassurance such as, 'It's nothing to worry about,'; reasoned arguments about the non-physical nature of the symptoms; doubts expressed as to the reality of the symptoms, such as, 'It's all in your mind,'; or invalidation of their experience, such as, 'People with x (an illness) don't get that.' Falling into one of these traps is not likely to help the patient. Nor will telling someone that in your view it is a marital problem, even if you are right! The therapist should only give relevant information and preferably the minimum necessary. It is essential to check that the patient has understood it in the way the therapist thought they had expressed it. Rather than reassure the patient that the symptom is not physical, the therapist can collaborate with them in trying to find out what might be happening. Finding out the patient's beliefs and working out ways of testing those with the patient may be a key task. Taking the opportunities presented within sessions, such as symptom appearance at moments of anxiety (perhaps over being late), can be extremely useful for exploring with the patient the role of thoughts, beliefs and anxiety.

There are several possible ways of intervening with patients complaining of physical symptoms for whom no organic diagnosis can be made. Apart from medication changes and alterations towards a more healthy lifestyle, it is possible to help people clarify and change their beliefs about their health and the feared outcome. This involves finding out how the patient came to these beliefs and helping them construct alternative explanations for their observations. For example, a patient may believe their headache to presage a stroke, rather than noticing that it occurs at times of increased tension, such as around the time of an extended visit from the much loved but rowdy grandchildren. It may be necessary to discuss the beliefs which have led them to alter their lifestyle in an attempt to protect themselves, such as spending time in bed with a headache, or to reduce symptoms, such as staying as immobile as possible to reduce joint pain, and which then lead to disabling restrictions to their lifestyle or to exacerbation of their condition or their worries.

It is important to clarify the role of reassurance with the patient, as repeated investigations or visits to the doctor may bring short-term relief, but patients may then ruminate over the reassurance given or the proposed investigation and find something that makes them even more anxious. Whatever the mechanism, the search for reassurance may become protracted. People sometimes suggest that relatives refuse to offer reassurance, but this is extremely difficult for the relative to resist and seems only to work where the patient can accept the point of the strategy.

Case history 6.2:

Mrs I.D. was a 69-year-old woman who presented with abdominal pains and a conviction these pains were the result of cancer. A depressive hypochondriasis was diagnosed and her response to mono-amine oxidase inhibitors was dramatic, but despite this she failed to take these anti-depressants on discharge and quickly relapsed. In addition to looking at the problem of compliance within therapeutic sessions, it was clear on discharge that she still had some erroneous beliefs regarding her health. Thus despite the GP weighing her regularly, she was convinced she was losing weight and hence had a serious illness. When she discovered the therapist was interested in finding out what was really happening, she readily agreed to a 'reality test'. Thus she was to self-monitor her own weight and bring the results in to each session for the therapist to record. As part of this, it was explained that she would need to use the same weighing machine, wear similar clothing, and to expect a two lb fluctuation because of fluid balance.

Within the space of three or four weeks she agreed that in fact she was not losing weight and was able to explore further how this belief and others like it, for example regarding her medication, could actually adversely affect her life. Eventually through becoming more socially active, she developed a close relationship with a man and was helped through some of her anxiety about becoming sexually active again for the first time since the death of her second husband. There were no further problems with medication compliance.

6.5.3 Techniques for anxiety reduction

Various factors may contribute to each elderly individual's health anxiety (see Figure 6.2). They must be identified and their relative importance evaluated. Information can be gathered from careful interviews with the elderly patient and perhaps also with involved family members or supporters. Where someone is reluctant or apparently unable to give much detail about their circumstances a great deal of information can sometimes be gathered by the detailed review of an average day, from waking up in the morning to going to bed at night. Noticing the effects of the symptoms on this average day can give information about what might be raising anxiety, how the patients cope with their symptoms and what kind of social contacts and interests they have.

Health anxiety can interact with symptoms, as for example raised anxiety can heighten the experience of pain. When the experience of pain also induces anxiety, there may result a self-maintaining loop: a vicious circle. Some people interpret the effects of physiological arousal as symptoms of illness. Figure 6.3 is a simplified model of hypochondriasis based on this idea. It can be seen, then, that reducing the elderly person's level of anxiety directly or indirectly will break this vicious circle and reduce the experience of physical symptoms, which should in

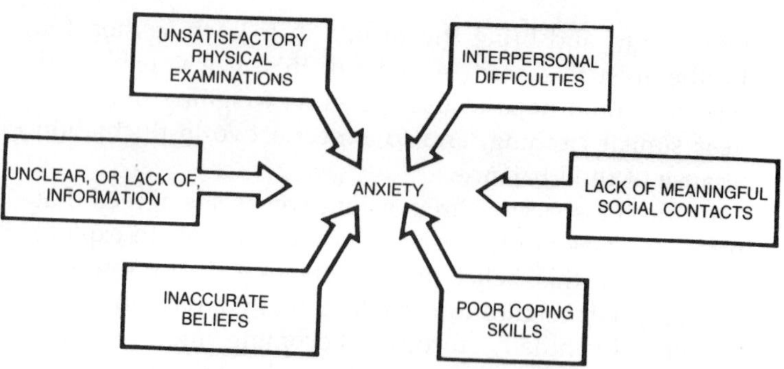

Figure 6.2 Factors exacerbating anxiety in the elderly person showing hypochondriasis.

turn lead to an abatement of the hypochondriacal complaints. For a more comprehensive approach to psychological strategies for pain, the reader is referred elsewhere [14].

For those patients whose symptoms are attributable to the physiological signs of anxiety, which are then seen as dangerous, techniques to control anxiety itself may prove helpful. Once again, the acceptability of the technique to the patient is of paramount importance, as most proponents of relaxation exercises stress the need for repeated practice. The most widely used technique still is probably progressive muscle relaxation. The procedure for this involves learning to discriminate better between tense and relaxed states of muscular tension, and increasing control over relaxation of key muscles [15]. As with all skills, it is harder to acquire when someone is in an acute state of anxiety but it may be useful with old people who have specific or less severe anxiety. An alternative method of relaxation which elderly people often find easier to use is autogenic training. In this, a pleasant image, such as lying on a beach on a warm summer's day, is brought vividly to mind, producing a feeling of calm. Pre-recorded cassettes may have some limited use, but are not a substitute for training in relaxation procedures with a professional experienced in teaching the methods, let alone a full psychological approach. In all cases, clear explanation, training in self-monitoring and a supportive, gradual approach will aid the development of relaxation skills.

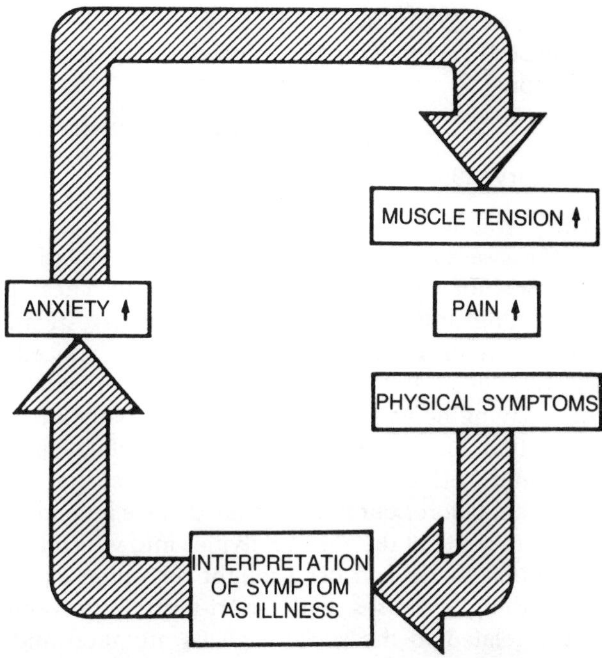

Figure 6.3 Simplified model of hypochondriasis illustrating the role of anxiety.

Breathing problems are common in old people, and some of these instances are psychogenic, that is, hyperventilation. This is characterized by shallow, thoracic, rapid breathing and has been shown to generate unpleasant physiological symptoms within the space of a few minutes [16, 17]. The appearance of these is often related to anxiety-laden or meaningful events or thoughts. One way of treating this is to facilitate relearning of a normal breathing pattern. This involves learning to slow the speed of breathing and use of the diaphragm rather than the upper chest.

Some people, elderly or not, find other techniques helpful, such as meditation, yoga and Tai Chi Chuan, and there seems no reason why these may not be beneficial. This last is a slow, flowing, dance-like series of movements. It involves learning to control breathing through the use of the diaphragm, and to use different muscle groups simultaneously without tensing other parts of the body, embodying the principles of correct breathing and relaxation.

Case history 6.3:

Mr G.M. was a sprightly widower in his seventies referred for assessment following repeated presentations at his doctor's for physical complaints, mainly chest pain and breathing difficulties. After numerous investigations and an operation for a condition he had not noticed but which had been found on examination, he still complained, saying he was worse than ever. Taking a history revealed that his symptoms had started while his wife was ill, and had been better at times since her death twelve years before, but had worsened since he had withdrawn from some of the social activities into which he had thrown himself. He had been taught relaxation exercises and breathing exercises with short-term improvement, probably related to the social aspects, attention and interest. Anti-depressant medication was not indicated. Anxieties about his future and loneliness were important factors in his situation. He was offered counselling sessions, in which the aim was explicitly to help him understand and cope with his life situation. For some time, he insisted on a medical view of his problems, and repeatedly sought further investigations, but eventually began to acknowledge the improvement that the sessions brought him. This led to a preparedness to consider the emotional aspects of his experience and he talked about his anxieties of being ill, dependent and isolated. For some time he was depressed as he regretted the loss of his wife and not finding another partner. His physical complaints became less important to him and he began to use the health services more appropriately.

In addition to relaxation procedures, there are techniques such as biofeedback, which enable a person to gain some control over physiological functioning through immediate feedback.

6.5.4 Relationship problems and interpersonal difficulties

As people age, they may become more dependent on their environment and on the people around them. They may have to adapt to reduced income, impaired mobility, both loss of physical fitness and transport, and changes in their social and family networks. The importance of increased dependence on family members or caring neighbours should not be underestimated. Younger people are much more able to remove themselves from unsatisfactory or distressing relationships or to find substitutes. They may also be in a position to exercise control over the terms of the relationship. Elderly people who are experiencing such distress in relationships may be unwilling or unable to remove themselves from the situation, and indeed may be dependent in some important way on the relationships they find difficult. For some, the dependence in itself may be distressing, particularly if the person has spent half a lifetime since childhood avoiding the experience.

Case history 6.4:

Mr N.K. had always been the dominant partner in his marriage, and made the decisions about household routine, holidays and interior decoration. His wife was rather timid and had looked up to and depended on her husband for many years, even to the extent that she rarely left the house without him. After his stroke, the couple had to change their routines. The balance of power within the relationship also had to change, with responsibility for money and dealings with outside agencies falling on Mrs N.K. This led to anxiety and resentment on her part, while Mr N.K. hated the position he found himself in and began to accuse her of taking money and deceiving him. Moreover, he refused to dress himself and frequently became distressed by thoughts of his condition and his future death. On referral, work with the couple proved difficult, but after a physical assessment, the team members focused on attempts to help Mr N.K. understand the nature of his condition, with help from an occupational therapist for assessment and aids. One team member saw

Mrs N.K. to provide support and encouragement for her attempts to develop her skills and an independent life, and to help her relate to her husband in a less critical way, but without falling in with his demands. Mr N.K. never accepted his condition with equanimity, but the couple managed to continue to live together.

In this case, a physical illness combined with health anxiety in a man who found it hard to tolerate illness and dependency, leading to increased demands for care from his wife.

On the other hand, an old person who suffers from a poor social network, a very low level of perceived emotional contact with important family members, or dissatisfaction with the quality of interaction, can find that the sick role brings with it a sudden and dramatic increase in time, concern and interest from others. Becoming 'well' again can mean a return to the previous unwanted situation. In a few instances visits from family members can be contingent only upon 'real' physical illness as the family do not believe in anxiety or depression, nor accept any role in the development or maintenance of distressing relationships.

Case history 6.5:

Mrs O.D., a 71-year-old widow, was referred some months after a heart attack, at the instigation of her son. Her GP had known her for many years and felt she had used illness as a means of controlling her family in the past. Mrs O.D. described herself as independent, and said she did not want to be a burden on her children. At the time of her heart attack, the family had rallied round, each of her three children visiting and contributing to her convalescence. When they attempted to go back to the normal routine, of weekly visits in one instance and less frequent calls from the other two children, both of whom lived some distance away, Mrs O.D. began to complain of dizziness and breathlessness. She said she was frightened that she would have another heart attack. These episodes occurred several times towards the end of visits, but also at other times, such as in the middle of the night and on

Sunday evenings. Reassurance from her doctor and the specialist did not help. On assessment, there was little reason to suspect that Mrs O.D. had any physical disability to explain her difficulties, but she was adamant that she could not undertake a range of activities, such as some household tasks and socializing at the Community Centre near where she lived, because she was afraid her symptoms would start. She was asked by the psychologist to keep a diary of her symptoms, and when they talked about their appearance, Mrs O.D. could see how they coincided with events she found stressful or upsetting. The psychologist talked further with her about the nature of anxiety and how its effects could be interpreted as similar to her earlier physical symptoms. It was clear that the symptoms were serving to keep Mrs O.D.'s children involved, and after some time it became possible to discuss with Mrs O.D. the cost of having her children visit under duress, along with the possible benefits of alternatives, mainly reinstating her friendships with her neighbours and the other residents in her complex. A graded series of exercises were agreed to allow Mrs O.D. to venture outside her home without too much initial anxiety, and once she was out her neighbours welcomed her back. Mrs O.D. stopped calling her children at night. She made a good friend of a new resident and her 'attacks' became of less importance as she began to enjoy her life again.

In this case, Mrs O.D. was able to use the input she was given, but in other cases the whole family may have to be involved in any intervention. A similar phenomenon can occur when a professional becomes involved; for example, one community nurse asked for help when a patient became worse every time he mentioned discharge. Eventually, he agreed to a prolonged contract with his patient but reduced the frequency of sessions over time, so that the patient felt less need to ensure his visits continued by complaining of symptoms. She also eventually improved in this respect with a change in her life circumstances.

In some instances, being ill may seem the only acceptable way to retain a dependent relationship.

Case history 6.6:

Mrs B.F. was referred to the team at the age of 69, three years after the death of her husband, suffering from depression and complaining that she was sufficiently ill that she could not look after herself. The event immediately prior to and precipitating referral was the diagnosis in her sister of heart disease. Mrs W.Y., her much younger sister of 52, lived nearby, and in addition to bringing up her teenage family, running a household and working part-time, she had cleaned Mrs B.F.'s house, done her shopping and washed her laundry. The diagnosis had led to Mrs W.Y. deciding she had to reduce unnecessary responsibilities and to look after herself better. Mrs B.F. had responded to the suggestion that she might take some of her household tasks back with increased demands and upset. On investigation, there seemed no medical reason why Mrs B.F. should not be completely independent. However, a history from herself and her sister suggested that Mrs B.F. had always been 'delicate' and had been 'spoiled' by her husband, who had done a great deal of the housework himself. For her part, Mrs B.F. had enjoyed working in their shop, but had never forgiven him for being retired and having to move them to another house. In a meeting arranged with two team members present to attempt to resolve the situation between the two sisters, Mrs W.Y. asserted her independence. Mrs B.F. was offered both home help and assistance in developing independent living skills. She accepted these reluctantly, but very soon after decided to enter a private Residential Home, where she enjoyed the company and the attendance.

6.6 ILLNESS BEHAVIOUR

Illness behaviour is a normal phenomenon. Each of us will react to illness in a variety of ways, depending on the nature of the symptoms, the immediate circumstances, our attitudes and beliefs. The behaviour and attitudes of others will also affect our behaviour. The sick role has certain benefits and costs. For example, if we are ill, others might treat us with tea and sympathy, or take over household tasks. If we have a high temperature, we might retreat to bed, but if we have to sit an important examination, miss our own birthday party or lose wages, we would probably soldier on. We each weigh up the pros and cons of going sick. For a person to take on a sick role needs the agreement of others. Norms for the sick role are based on cultural and social conventions and are partially learned within the family. Some people behave in unusual ways, that are thought by others to be abnormal. To outsiders, the behaviour may seem irrational, selfish or destructive.

The individuals who are referred because of the problems that adopting the sick role causes for themselves and others present a complex set of problems to those trying to help them. These problems may include the need to understand the gains and losses for the particular person at this time, in the particular circumstances. It may be necessary to understand the gains and losses for others involved with the person who is using the sick role. The responses of others may be crucial in the maintenance or improvement of these difficulties. For example, one study of married chronic pain patients showed that a reduction of attention by the spouses to their pain behaviour resulted in significantly lower levels of reported pain [18]. The relationship between events, symptoms and behaviours may be hard to elucidate. Changing a long-standing pattern of behaviours and interactions may be extremely difficult [19].

One of the most important aims of any treatment plan is to enable the person to satisfy their needs in a way that is acceptable to themselves and others. For example, if the sick role is adopted because it is the only apparent means for gaining visits from the family, then visits from the family may need to be arranged under other conditions. If this is just not possible, then acceptable alternative sources of company and attention may need to be sought. Often, it is difficulty in satisfying just this kind of ordinary human need that leads to behaviours that are considered by others to be manipulative. Using the sick role to control others without facing arguments or the anxiety of asserting oneself is also a possible motive to consider. If such factors are important, then it may be possible to facilitate changes through encouraging the development of social skills, or through marital or family work.

Facilitating self-help behaviour is a common problem where there is little self-help behaviour to start with and it is tempting for relatives, with only a limited amount of time, to do household tasks. There is often a pressure to take over tasks as a sign of caring. One common constellation of problems concerns the couple who find they have difficulties adjusting to retirement. When the woman becomes ill, the couple find a satisfactory resolution to their difficulties in the adoption of a pattern in which she remains an invalid, while her husband takes over the running of the house. Finally, some relatives become upset to see the patient perform tasks slowly or inefficiently and may find it hard to stand back and do nothing.

Case history 6.7:

Mrs C.F. was a 77-year-old divorced woman living on her own who was visited three or four times a week by her caring stepdaughter. Mrs C.F.'s husband, who had left her a number of years previously because of her illness behaviour, lived nearby and had developed dementia. She had a long history of taking to her bed as a means of coping and indeed, during her marriage, a housekeeper had been employed because of her failure to take on this role. She was diagnosed as having a neurotic depression and the community nurse asked the clinical psychologist to become involved because of difficulty in being able to help. Because of the resentment shown by Mrs C.F. to the community nurse and psychiatrist, and the high level of care and involvement shown by the stepdaughter, it was decided that it might be more constructive and effective to decide on a treatment plan which the stepdaughter could carry out. She had already developed a planned week which involved sharing her time between her stepmother, father, own family and part-time job! She was particularly concerned at what she regarded as the wasted life her stepmother was leading and how her preoccupation with her physical state had driven away most remaining social contacts. The stepdaughter was extremely pleased to have a specific plan to work from as she felt she never knew

Table 6.3 Mrs C.F.'s problems and treatment approach

Problem	*Solution*
Resents visit by psychiatrist/ psychologist	Intervene through caring stepdaughter
Constant talk about physical state	Reduce time and input associated with this
Little normal conversation	Time and interest increased when this produced
Infrequent self and house-care activity	Increase encouragement or reinforcement for attempts
Lack of insight about constant talk of physical symptoms	When complaints above a certain level, stepdaughter leaves, after explaining reason why
Suicidal/severe illness behaviour, e.g. heart attack, phone calls at 2.00 a.m.	Stepdaughter visits stepmother but limits stay to one minute if no evidence of illness

how best to cope with her stepmother's behaviour. The main points of the plan are presented in Table 6.3 and it involved her redistributing her time and care to reinforce more appropriate aspects of her stepmother's behaviour. A further aim was to reduce the antagonism which the stepmother's behaviour generated in the stepdaughter. Thus the stepdaughter was given verbal strategies which allowed her to state clearly her care for her stepmother, even in the most annoying situations such as a middle-of-the-night call-out, without reinforcing these aspects of her stepmother's behaviour. Over a six-week period on a 10-point rating scale (with 10 representing the worst illness behaviour and 0 representing acceptable illness behaviour) the stepdaughter's average rating per week changed from 7.5 to 5.0, indicating a definite improvement. This was further confirmed by a visit two months later by the psychiatrist who found her mental state 'much improved'. This improvement continued through to follow-up nine months later, even though the stepdaughter had to reduce the time spent with her stepmother because of her father's increasing confusion and disability. It is interesting that behavioural change took place more slowly than the change in Mrs C.F.'s verbal behaviour. Thus the stepdaughter noticed her stepmother talking less about her physical state and being aware of and stopping herself in mid-stream of physical complaints saying to the step-daughter, for example, 'But you don't want to hear about that, do you,' prior to her taking up various household tasks again.

6.7 SERVICE CONSIDERATIONS

6.7.1 Communication and education

It is perhaps unfortunate that it is so difficult to use strategies for understanding health anxieties and illness behaviours. Our health services are set up with discrete physical illness in mind and strongly reinforce the presentation of complaints of physical symptoms. Medical staff time and interventions are only offered on presentation of symptoms. Both patient and medical staff wish for and are happiest with a clear diagnosis of an easily treatable physical illness. The patient may be punitive towards the doctor who dares suggest an alternative, psychological rationale. Given that some patients may present with different complaints over the years, it is hard to know when there is sufficient evidence of a strong psychological component, and yet there are patients who have undergone several serious and costly investigations that were totally unnecessary and even harmful, because they are determined that the cause of their distress is physical disease. The earlier identification of such patients by those working both in psychiatry and general medicine could lead to better treatment.

In addition, it should not be forgotten that physical illness may be an important factor in distress. Families may join with an individual in attempting to find satisfactory solutions to life's problems. Some of these attempts may bring additional problems, while the need to deal with social and medical structures can demand enormous persistence, patience and ingenuity [20]. Educating the psychiatric team in developing a common understanding and approach towards particular problems such as this is an important task in developing true multidisciplinary team work. In addition, communication across service boundaries and education of health professionals may in the long term make for improved practice.

6.7.2 Coping with persistent complaints

The elderly person who has shown a life-long pattern of illness complaints, and who may often be taking a number of inappropriate and possibly harmful medicines, presents particular difficulties for the health services. These patients have often either failed to respond to traditional physical psychiatric treatments, or refused to have anything to do with psychiatry because of the stigma and because they believe their problems are physical! It can be almost impossible to discover what psychological factors were present 30 or 40 years ago to cause the problem to develop.

It has been the aim throughout this chapter to present a realistic account of the challenges facing a team working with this particular clinical group. Even so, it may be argued that we have erred on the side of being too optimistic about the prognosis of elderly people presenting with anxieties about their health. However, there have been recent developments within health psychology which are useful in the understanding and treatment of such difficulties.

Even with the most effective use of models and skills, there are some people with hypochondriacal complaints whom it is impossible to help. In these cases it is worth remembering Figure 6.3 which indicates that any increased anxiety is likely to exacerbate the hypochondriacal behaviour. It is then important for the practitioners involved to minimize any additional anxiety that they contribute. An example follows in Table 6.4 of a strategy which might be used to try to cope with an elderly person who phones the GP's surgery ten times a week complaining of serious illnesses, along with the rationale for each part of the plan. Similar plans can be drawn up to cope with patients who hound the doctor or nurse on the ward, or who talk incessantly about their symptoms and not themselves. Providing such a clear structure may not be a cure, but helps to limit the damage patients do to themselves, opens the way to improvement and may reduce the stress felt by the professionals involved by giving them a coping strategy.

Table 6.4 Example of a plan for use with hypochondriacal patient who rings the GP surgery ten times per week for home consultations

1. One regular visit per week (not following a call). To include five minutes' physical examination and firm reassurance. This ensures the need is met independent of the telephone calls, which are less strongly reinforced.
2. Whenever possible, only one named GP to provide consultations (the GP who is most willing to see the client). This provides consistency and enables the doctor to keep track of the situation.
3. An extra visit is carried out if two days pass without any phone call from patient (criteria to be altered if situation improves). This reinforces not telephoning.
4. If GP has to respond to a 'false' urgent call, e.g. patient feigning heart attack, visit should be conducted in a calm manner, examination should be the minimum necessary to exclude a real medical emergency and should be time limited, i.e. five minutes or less. The GP should leave as soon as possible with a brief informative comment to patient (e.g. 'You are not suffering from a heart attack, I have to leave now,'). The information is minimal to avoid unnecessary reinforcement of the behaviour, and to give the least possible grounds for misunderstanding.
5. GP's staff are given precise instructions as to what information to give during phone calls by patient. This again reduces potential reinforcement and allows for the minimum possible misinterpretation.

6.8 CONCLUSION

In this chapter the range of psychiatric diagnoses has been described and considerations for assessment and physical treatment has been discussed as well as some of the psychological models available for understanding health anxiety and other health-related problems. Some pointers for treatment have also been mentioned. Medical and psychological approaches are complementary rather than exclusive in nature. Neglecting either is likely to lead to an ineffective intervention. Developing effective care for elderly people with such problems will depend on the ability of those professionals involved to develop a model and a way of working collaboratively acceptable to them all.

REFERENCES

1. World Health Organization (1992) *The ICD10 Classification of Mental and Behavioural Disorders.* World Health Organization, Geneva.
2. Kenyon, F.E. (1964) Hypochondriasis: a clinical study. *British Journal of Psychiatry*, **110**, 478–88.
3. Wilson, L.A., Lawson, I.R. and Brass, H. (1962) Multiple disorders in the elderly. *Lancet*, **2**, 841–3.
4. De Alaracon, R. (1964) Hypochondriasis and depression in the aged. *Gerontologia Clinica*, **6**, 266–77.
5. Bradley, J.J. (1963) Severe localised pain associated with depressive syndrome. *British Journal of Psychiatry*, **109**, 741–5.
6. Webb, H.E. and Lascelle, R.G. (1962) Treatment of facial and head pain associated with depression. *Lancet*, **1**, 355.
7. Barskey, A.J. and Klerman, G.L. (1983) Overview: hypochondriasis, bodily complaints and somatic styles. *American Journal of Psychiatry*, **140**, 273–81.
8. Lacks, P. (1987) *Behavioural Treatment for Persistent Insomnia*, Pergamon, New York.
9. Roth, P.M., Caron, M.S., Ort, R.S. *et al.* (1962) Patient's beliefs about peptic ulcer and its treatment. *Annals of Internal Medicine*, **56**, 72–80.
10. Trethowan, W.H. (1983) Pain in the mind. *The Midland Journal of Psychotherapy*, **1**, 56–64.
11. Kellner, R. (1986) *Somatization and Hypochondriasis*, Praeger, New York.
12. Hawton, K., Salkovskis, P.M., Kirk, J. and Clark, D.M. (1989) *Cognitive Behaviour Therapy for Psychiatric Problems: a Practical Guide*, Oxford University Press, Oxford.
13. Salkovskis, P.M. (1989) Somatic problems, in *Cognitive Behaviour Therapy for Psychiatric Problems: a Practical Guide*, (eds K. Hawton, P.M. Salkovskis, J. Kirk and D.M. Clark), Oxford University Press, Oxford.
14. Philips, H.C. (1988) *The Psychological Management of Chronic Pain: a Manual*. Springer, New York.
15. Rimm, D.C. and Masters, J.C. (1974) *Behaviour Therapy: Techniques and Empirical Findings*, Academic Press, London.
16. Ley, R. (1985) Agoraphobia, the panic attack and the hyperventilation syndrome. *Behaviour Research and Therapy*, **23**(1), 79–82.
17. Lum, L.C. (1976) The syndrome of habitual hyperventilation, in *Modern Trends in Psychosomatic Medicine*, Volume 3, (ed. O. Hill), Butterworth, London.
18. Block, A.R., Kremer, E.F., and Gaylor, M. (1980) Behavioural treatment of chronic pain: the spouse as a discriminative cue for pain behaviour, *Pain*, **9**, 243–52.
19. Wooley, S.C., Blackwell, B., and Winget, C. (1978) A learning

theory model of chronic illness behaviour, treatment and research. *Psychosomatic Medicine*, **40**(5), 379–401.

20. Anderson, R. and Bury, M. (eds) (1988) *Living with Chronic Illness: the Experience of Patients and their Families*, Unwin Hyman, London.

7

Hallucinations, delusions and persecutory states

Hallucinations, delusions and persecutory phenomena often go hand-in-hand. When we consider the human need to explain and make sense of a situation, this is perhaps not surprising. Someone who has an inexplicable sensory experience may well find an explanation in a persecutory delusion. Despite the frequent interaction of hallucinations, delusions and persecutory states, they are not always related. For clarity, we will therefore first deal with hallucinations and then consider separately delusions and persecutory phenomena.

7.1 HALLUCINATIONS

The type of hallucination may be a guide to diagnosis. Auditory hallucinations are found most commonly in schizophrenia, although they sometimes also occur in affective illness, when the content is consonant with the patient's depressed or elevated mood. Hearing one's thoughts spoken out loud or hearing two voices discussing one in the third person were, along with other so-called 'first-rank' symptoms of schizophrenia, often regarded as diagnostic of schizophrenia. In old age, these symptoms have been correlated with changes in cortical structure [1]. Visual hallucinations, on the other hand, are generally regarded as the hallmark of organic states, especially acute confusional states. Perhaps the best known of these are the vivid visual hallucinations of alcohol withdrawal ('delirium tremens', ICD10; F10.4) which can occur in other drug-withdrawal states.

Case history 7.1:

Mrs D.F. was an 83-year-old widow with poor eyesight living alone but near her son. She had been on lorazepam for many years, and fell, fracturing her femur. In hospital she made a good recovery from the operation, but then seemed to become depressed. Her lorazepam was stopped, and an anti-depressant started. Over the next few days she became much more disturbed, and one night believed that she had wakened to see her son being dismembered. For several days she was convinced that he had, in fact, been murdered. A benzodiazepine was re-started, and the problems resolved though she remained apprehensive about being discharged.

This lady illustrates the complexities of medical care for old people. Her fall may have been precipitated by poor eyesight and medication. The subsequent visual hallucination was probably related to benzodiazepine withdrawal, poor eyesight, and possibly to the anti-cholinergic effect of the anti-depressant. Change of environment, pain and analgesics may also have played a part. Relative sensory deprivation through poor eyesight and hearing are important contributory factors for hallucinations and paranoid states. The relationship between poor hearing and persecutory states has long been recognized [2], though a study of patients attending a hearing clinic found that depression was the problem most frequently associated with hearing loss [3]. Sometimes impaired sight may produce a frightening hallucinosis without associated persecutory phenomena: the Charles Bonnet syndrome.

Case history 7.2:

Miss K.B. was an 87-year-old lady who, although severely handicapped by arthritis, lived in her own back-to-back terraced house. She suffered visual hallucinations which developed in complexity over a six-week period until she saw images of cats in her bedroom, a number seven bus going across her sitting-room ceiling and a man building a glass box in the corner. These hallucinations were of normal size and colour and became more apparent in the evening and night-time. They were only in one sensory modality. The patient was intellectually intact on brief testing and perplexed and frightened by her experience. The psychiatrist started her on a small dose of thioridazine as symptomatic treatment and arranged further investigations. An investigation by a neurologist into the possibility of temporal lobe seizures (TLE) was negative and drew the unhelpful comment, 'I imagine these are just delusions of the senile brain.' A detailed neuropsychological investigation showed the patient was intellectually well-preserved with good insight into her condition. An EEG (electroencephalogram) was arranged but the patient refused this, mainly because of embarrassment as she was bald and wore a wig! Her hallucinations were not stereotyped and there was nothing else to suggest TLE so we concluded that the hallucinations were due to sensory deprivation.The psychologist reassured her and explained her hallucinations to her as an unusual but well-recognized complication of failing eyesight (known as the Charles Bonnet syndrome). The thioridazine was discontinued. The hallucinations continued but the patient did not find them so troublesome. She eventually confided that she had put off seeking help for several weeks because she was afraid she was going mad.

Other types of hallucination, e.g. touch (tactile) and smell (olfactory), are rarer in old age. Tactile hallucinations of a sexual kind are sometimes found in paraphrenic schizophrenia (ICD10; F20, Paranoid schizophrenia). The content of an hallucination can also help in diagnosis. Hallucinations consistent with a poor self-image, for example, voices accusing the patient of acts of which she believes she is guilty, or hallucinations that the patient smells, linked perhaps with the delusions that she is dirty, are often associated with a severely depressed mood. Not all hallucinations in depressive disorder have an obviously depressive interpretation for the patient. Sometimes hallucinations of voices saying unpleasant things about the patient are felt to be unjustified and are interpreted in a persecutory way.

Associated findings such as poor eyesight or hearing or acute physical illness can help in diagnosis and management. One condition in which mentally well people sometimes experience apparent auditory or visual hallucinations is following bereavement (see Chapter 4).

The commonest cause of predominantly visual hallucinations in old age is an organic brain disorder [4], often delirium, but sometimes dementia, especially of the vascular type and, possibly, diffuse Lewy-body dementia. The role of medication, and drug withdrawal (especially from benzodiazepines), in precipitating delirium must be stressed. The commonest cause of predominantly auditory hallucinations is **paranoid schizophrenia** (F20.0), though depressive disorders and bereavement reactions also account for a proportion. The core symptoms of paranoid schizophrenia are delusions, often persecutory, hallucinatory voices that threaten or instruct the patient and hallucinations of smell, taste, sexual or other bodily sensation. Thought disorder is more commonly found in earlier-onset forms of schizophrenia. Visual and hearing impairment are important in increasing an elderly person's susceptibility to hallucination, regardless of diagnosis. In temporal lobe epilepsy, stereotyped hallucinations may occur, sometimes in several modalities. Figure 7.1 provides a flow chart to help the diagnosis of hallucinations.

7.2 DELUSIONS

These persistent false beliefs, incompatible with the individual's cultural and educational background, are found in fragmentary form in **delirium**. They are, however, more characteristic of **paranoid schizophrenia** (F20.0) or **delusional disorders** (F22.0). The latter group of disorders is characterized by the development either of a single delusion or of a group of related delusions, without predominant hallucinations. There is considerable overlap of phenomenology and response to neuroleptic treatment between delusional disorder and paranoid schizophrenia. Delusions that a patient has an incurable illness, that she has committed some terrible crime and others of a similar kind occur in **severe depressive episodes** (e.g. F32.3). Occasionally these delusions may be of a persecutory nature, for example that she is about to be evicted from her house,

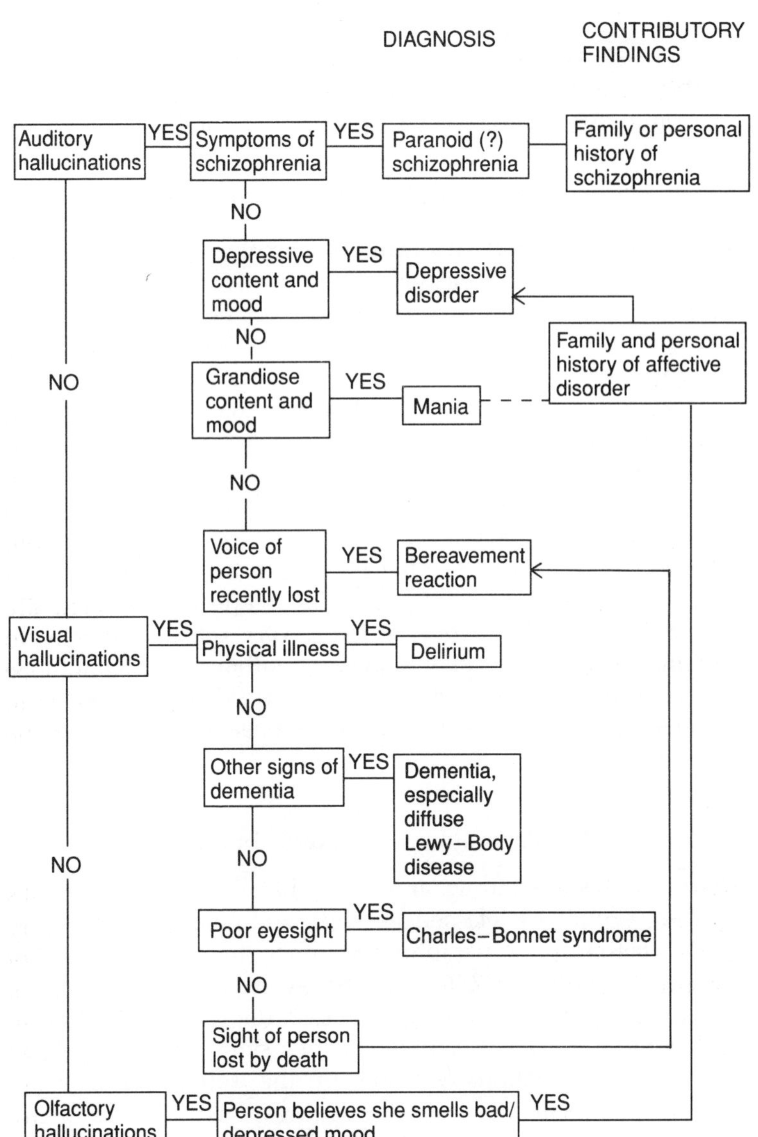

Figure 7.1 Flow chart for the diagnosis of hallucinations.

though even then it may be possible to find a link with the lack of self-esteem or guilt associated with depressed mood (perhaps she thinks the eviction is because of some crime she has committed).

7.3 PERSECUTORY STATES

We admire children for their innocence but go to great pains to teach them to be suspicious of the motives of others, first through fairy tales and then through specific warnings not to take sweets from, or go with strangers. Because there are unscrupulous people who will exploit or harm vulnerable children or old people, we have to encourage a certain amount of suspiciousness. Some people take this necessary caution too far, and become suspicious of all outsiders. People with such a personality (**paranoid personality disorder**, F60.0) may develop an isolated, self-sufficient lifestyle which enables them to avoid warm social contact with other people. In old age, physical or psychiatric illness suddenly puts them in a position where they do need outside help, but find this very difficult to accept. Organic brain disease may supervene either coincidentally or as a consequence of a restricted or bizarre diet. Alternatively, a frank paranoid schizophrenia or delusional disorder may develop.

7.3.1 Paranoid schizophrenia in old age

There has been a strong argument that the term 'late paraphrenia' should be retained for this syndrome in old age [5]. ICD10 classifies 'late paraphrenia' under the syndrome of **delusional disorder** (F22.0), but the syndrome defined operationally by Roth [6] as a late-onset disorder characterized by 'a well organised system of paranoid delusions with or without auditory hallucinations existing in the setting of a well-preserved personality and affective response' obviously includes some cases that would be classified by ICD10 as paranoid schizophrenia. Some writers have further complicated the situation by failing to separate this disorder from organic paranoid states.

The history of the concept of late paraphrenia is discussed in detail by Grahame [7] in a paper which argues firmly in favour of retaining this diagnosis. Late paraphrenia develops in people, usually women, of a paranoid or schizoid premorbid personality. They are usually single, or have had unsatisfactory marriages and sexual adjustment, perhaps related to sexual abuse in childhood. They have few or no surviving children, and are often chronically hard of hearing. People of lower social class seem to be more vulnerable, and sufferers often live in substandard inner-city housing. First-admission rates for schizophrenia peak in young adulthood but, especially for women, there is a further peak in those over 75 years old. This may reflect the influence of non-dementing organic brain damage, of sensory deprivation, or of increasing stresses as the capacity for independent living is compromised by physical or other psychiatric problems. Community prevalence is probably less than one per cent and it is seen less frequently in elderly inpatients with increasing sophistication in the use of neuroleptic drugs, including depot medication, to keep patients functioning relatively well in the community. Feelings of depressed mood are not uncommon in old people with paraphrenia, although the depression is almost invariably seen by the patient as a reaction to perceived wrongs, just as depressed patients with hypochondriacal symptoms often attribute their depression to supposed physical illness. The presence of paranoid symptoms in some patients suffering from moderate depressive illness can lead to difficulties in diagnosis. Schizoid or paranoid premorbid personality is a useful diagnostic pointer for paraphrenia whereas a personal or family history of affective disorder usually, though not invariably, points to a depressive diagnosis.

Case history 7.3:

Mrs B.K. was a 78-year-old widow who lived alone in an eighth floor high-rise flat. When seen at home she was, she said, feeling depressed and thought this might be due to the attentions paid her by a man at the Day Centre she attended. There were no clear hallucinations or delusions but the patient seemed cognitively slowed and preoccupied. The psychiatrist thought this might be evidence of a subtly varying level of awareness and arranged admission with a provisional diagnosis of early dementia, possibly of metabolic origin. On the ward, the patient developed a delusional conviction that another (male) patient was following her, and wanted to get into bed with her. She had auditory hallucinations of a voice telling her what to do and believed that her hands were being moved by an outside influence. The diagnosis of paraphrenia was made and she was treated successfully with trifluoperazine. No metabolic abnormalities were detected.

Late paraphrenia and related disorders respond well to treatment with neuroleptics, provided the patient can be persuaded to take them. Building a therapeutic relationship with an elderly paraphrenic person is often difficult but community nurses who usually give depot neuroleptic preparations to these patients are often adept. Often a compromise has to be worked out in terms of dosage such that patients' symptoms are controlled sufficiently for them to carry on with everyday life without excessive side-effects and with a minimum need for anti-cholinergic anti-Parkinsonian drugs which can themselves cause confusion. When depressive features persist despite adequate neuroleptic medication, anti-depressant medication or ECT can be added depending on circumstances.

7.3.2 Symptomatic paranoid states

(a) Mood disorder

Paranoid symptoms are not uncommon in moderately depressed old people. Post [8] has discussed the mixture of schizophrenic and affective symptoms in old age. He has also described a state of 'intermediate psychotic depression' [9] in which paranoid phenomena are relatively common and do not always have the characteristic that the patient believes the persecution is justified.

Case history 7.4:

A 72-year-old widow lived in a very poor back-to-back house with her daughter who suffered from severe obsessive compulsive disorder. The old lady was admitted to hospital with a severe psychotic depressive episode which was initially treated with anti-depressants. When she went home to the very restrictive life imposed by the daughter (who, incidentally, refused treatment for her own condition), she relapsed rapidly and had to be readmitted. She was so severely disabled that, on this occasion, she had to be given electro-convulsive therapy (ECT). She made a stormy recovery and for a period became quite paranoid, believing that we were experimenting on her and that we wanted to get rid of her. She eventually returned to good health and with maintenance antidepressant therapy, strong social support in the home and day-hospital attendance, she has remained well for a considerable time.

This case not only illustrates the way in which paranoid symptoms may form part of the symptom-picture of a depressed patient, it also illustrates how a patient can go through stages of depression during recovery. The daughter's severe obsessional neurosis also raises the question of a familial link between depressive illness and severe obsessional phenomena. This is not the only family in which we have seen severe obsessional phenomena in the child of a patient with mood disorder, and a higher frequency of schizophrenia has also been reported in the children of those with severe mood disorder. In old-age psychiatry, one often has the benefit not only of an antecedent family history, but also of a family history of mental illness in the patient's children. This can be diagnostically helpful, but sometimes it seems to call into question purist views of the genetics of mental illness.

Case history 7.5:

Mrs L.H. was a 75-year-old widow, admitted with an episode of hypomania following a move to an old person's home. She had a history of manic-depressive illness. On this occasion her mood was euphoric and she had slight pressure of ideas. She had ideas of reference and thought that a 'type of shock' was being imposed on her body.

After treatment, she returned to independent living in a new flat. Despite day-hospital support, she had six further admissions over a two-year period. On some occasions there was an element of manipulation in her admissions but most times there was also clear evidence of depressive episode. She also developed a severe anaemia, probably of dietary origin, which responded to treatment. On one occasion she became very suspicious, accusing us of treating her as a 'guinea pig'. Subsequently she remained relatively well at home on a tricyclic anti-depressant with support from a community nurse and a social worker as well as day-hospital and Day-Centre attendance.

This patient who normally had recurrent depressive episodes thus had a hypomanic episode with marked paranoid features. When severe persecutory phenomena occur in depressive illness or hypomania, it is fully justified to treat them in their own right with a neuroleptic; though neuroleptic treatment should never be continued indefinitely without good indication because of the risks of extra-pyramidal side-effects, especially tardive dyskinesia.

(b) Alcohol and drug abuse and dependence

An isolated **auditory hallucinosis** (ICD10; F10.52) or a full-blown **schizophreniform illness** (F10.50) can develop in elderly as well as younger alcohol abusers. **Alcohol withdrawal** (F10.3–10.4) can give rise to a state of irritability and even delirium with an affect of terror and frank persecutory phenomena. Withdrawal from barbiturates or benzodiazepines can also be responsible (F13.3–13.4).

Case history 7.6:

Mr J.H. was a 71-year-old widower, admitted via the casualty department with 'delirium'. Despite this, he was able to give a reasonably coherent history and his memory was only minimally impaired. About a week later he suddenly became very agitated and reported odd experiences. He believed he was working a four-on-four-off shift system and said he had to go to the graveyard. He absconded in the night to one of the other wards where he tried to drag two ladies out of bed. He had to be sedated and it was only subsequently that we found he had been abusing barbiturates at home. His delirium had some paranoid features and was probably due to barbiturate withdrawal.

Whenever a patient develops unexpected disturbed behaviour and persecutory symptoms within a week or so of admission, the possibility of drug or alcohol withdrawal should be investigated. Withdrawal states can generally be avoided by carefully planned withdrawal, if necessary with the use of a decreasing dosage regime of a sedative, non-epileptogenic drug like chlormethiazole. Long-standing abuse of amphetamines can also cause a schizophreniform psychosis (F15.5). Psychoses arising from drug abuse can be treated symptomatically (usually in hospital) while the offending drug is withdrawn

(c) Temporal lobe epilepsy

Although this is not specifically a condition of old age, it is worth noting that long-standing temporal lobe epilepsy can give rise to a schizophreniform psychosis [10]. Temporal lobe epilepsy itself can be associated with stereotyped and sometimes complex hallucinations.

(d) Delirium (acute confusional states)

Drug-withdrawal states are really a special form of delirium. There are many other causes of delirium (see Chapter 5). Fragmentary persecutory ideas and visual and auditory hallucinations may occur and the perplexed patient may react violently to those trying to help. Nursing in a well-lighted environment, with a regular nurse with the patient as much of the time as possible, will help. Continuing reassurance and re-orientation to take account of the patient's temporarily impaired mood and memory should be offered and will do a great deal to improve the patient's co-operation with essential physical treatment. Occasionally, neuroleptic treatment is justified, though, if there is a serious risk of provoking epileptic fits, a non-epileptogenic sedative such as chlormethiazole may be preferred.

(e) Dementia

Transient persecutory phenomena, particularly accusations that mislaid objects have been stolen, are a common part of early dementia. They do not usually merit treatment in their own right. Sometimes, especially in vulnerable personalities, the paranoid symptoms may cause serious problems for friends, neighbours or helping services. In these cases, symptomatic treatment with a neuroleptic such as low-dose haloperidol or thioridazine may be justified and will often produce improvement. Very occasionally a depot neuroleptic may be needed but the dose must be kept very small in view of the increased risk of accumulation and extra-pyramidal side-effects.

Case history 7.7:

Mrs S.C. was a 68-year-old widow who was estranged from her step-children. She had been married three times. She divorced her first husband, her second died suddenly and she was separated from her third. She developed the delusional belief that her third husband was coming into her flat secretly and moving furniture around. She suspected her neighbour of complicity in these plots. She had auditory hallucinations of her dead husband saying her name and believed she was 'clairvoyant'. She had minimal cognitive impairment (9/10 on the AMT) and the initial diagnosis was of paraphrenia. She was managed on neuroleptics as an inpatient initially, then as a day patient. She was also found to have cryptogenic fibrosing alveolitis (a lung condition). She was admitted to a medical ward following a collapse with a presumptive diagnosis of stroke: her paranoid ideas had abated but she appeared confused and her memory was impaired (AMT 6/10). After gradual improvement she returned home but six months later was readmitted with confusion and depressed mood. She was also said to be stripping off and going naked in her flat and to be neglecting herself. Her paranoid symptoms had disappeared but, in addition to slightly increased memory problems, she also had marked visuospatial dysfunction and neuro-psychological evaluation revealed clear evidence of organic involvement. Neuroleptics were stopped without recurrence of her paranoid symptoms or improvement in her cognitive state. After another period of day-hospital care she finally consented to go into residential care. She liked this and settled well. What initially appeared to be a paraphrenic illness was probably a paranoid reaction to memory problems associated with early multi-infarct dementia, although the possibility that she suffered from two distinct but coincidental psychiatric disorders cannot be ruled out.

This case illustrates how difficult diagnosis can be and how helpful it can be to a patient to have a specialist service involved in management over a protracted period of time.

Figure 7.2 is a flow chart which summarizes the main differential diagnosis of paranoid phenomena.

7.4 MANAGEMENT

7.4.1 Prevention

Sensory impairment and social isolation are important in all types of persistent persecutory states of late life. Deafness is usually long standing and early detection and prescription of aids may be helpful. On the other hand, many paranoid elderly people deliberately turn off their hearing-aids to limit contact with the outside world, so efforts in this direction may sometimes be wasted. Social isolation may even have a protective effect against the development of frank paranoid symptoms. Nevertheless, isolation should at least be seen as a risk factor for the development of paranoid illness or other conditions, and health and social services should keep a particularly close, though unobtrusive, watch on this vulnerable group. If simple isolation seems to be developing into paranoid schizophrenia or delusional disorder, then sympathetic but firm early intervention is required.

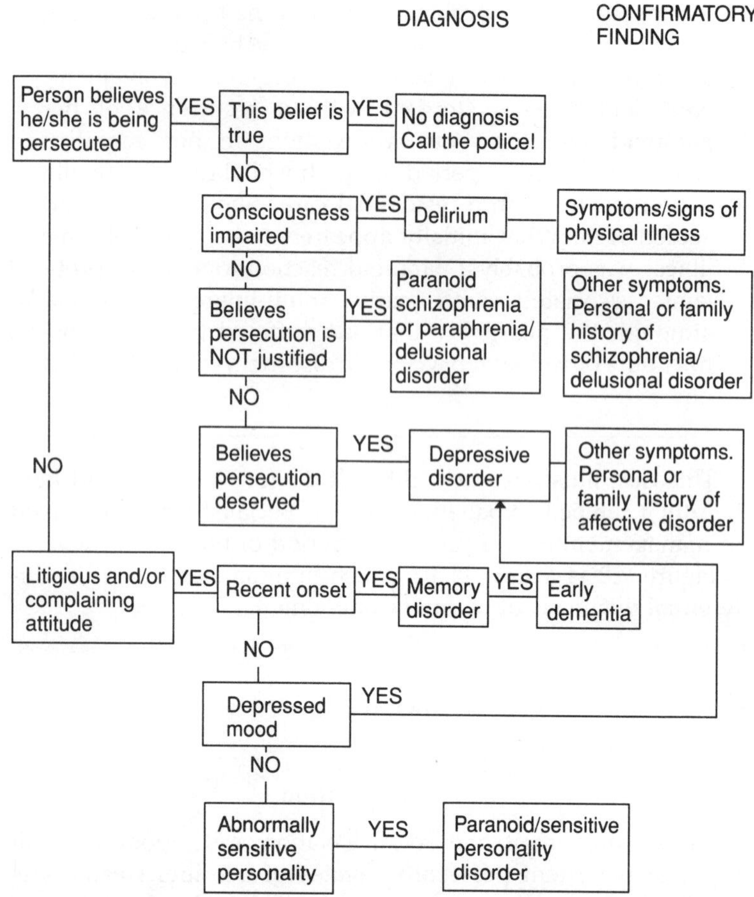

Figure 7.2 Flow chart for the diagnosis of persecutory states.

7.4.2 A personal approach

An accurate diagnosis is essential and this discussion presupposes that any medically treatable condition such as paraphrenia or physical illness has been diagnosed and treated. The major task for the therapeutic team is often to persuade the patient to accept help. If a specialist opinion is called for, whenever possible the specialist should be introduced to the patient by a person with whom the patient has a reasonable relationship (often the home-care worker or general practitioner). A key worker should be appointed as early as possible in the management of the case. It will be this person's task to win the confidence of the old person as far as possible. An understanding approach which respects the patient's need for social distance often works best. If memory is impaired, the patient may well still remember the visitor's face and whether its last appearance was pleasant or unpleasant! The first few contacts with the key worker should be used for getting to know the patient rather than persuading her to accept a particular line of treatment or to come into hospital. If hospital admission is essential for an unwilling patient (e.g. in the acutely disturbed paraphrenic patient), then this should be organized by the general practitioner and the specialist who made the assessment visit using compulsory powers if necessary. The key worker should be kept out of this as far as possible. Patients with paranoid symptoms often evoke responses which feed the paranoia. Helpers start to conceal information from the patient because they fear a paranoid reaction. A real incongruence between the expressed ideas and affect of the helpers may then be experienced by the paranoid patient 'confirming' his or her distrust of others [11]. Thus the patient's initial suspiciousness and (perhaps) delusions induce covert organized action and conspiratorial behaviour in others, confirming the original suspicion! Honest communication is important. Some strategies originally devised for dealing with 'confused talk' in patients with dementia, taken from a book on reality orientation [12] are useful and are summarized in Table 7.1.

Table 7.1 Strategies for dealing with confused talk

1. Tactfully disagree (on less sensitive subjects), or
2. Change the subject – discuss something more concrete, or
3. Acknowledge the feelings expressed – ignore the content.

(Source: Holden and Woods (1988) [12])

These strategies are relevant whether the patient is confused or not. The last is especially useful since it validates the patient's experience without colluding with the delusion or hallucination. One should avoid confirming delusions 'for the sake of a quiet life' but one should also avoid confrontation over delusions which will only lead to further entrenchment. Above all, one should always be scrupulously honest and open with paranoid patients. They will usually respect an honest communication, even if they disagree with it.

7.4.3 Medication

Fortunately, most hallucinatory and paranoid states show some response to neuroleptic medication. Where there is organic brain disease, however, the balance between the anti-psychotic effects of the drugs and unwanted side-effects is often difficult to achieve. Neuroleptic drugs are often cumulative in old age, and dosage regimes need to be monitored and often changed. Generally, one aims to keep the dose of the neuroleptic as low as possible rather than introducing anti-cholinergic, anti-Parkinsonian drugs which may themselves precipitate confusion. Drug treatment is discussed further in Chapter 9.

7.5 CONCLUSION

Hallucinations, delusions or persecutory phenomena are found in old-age mental illness of all types, often in association with sensory impairment. They are most consistently found in developed form in the late-onset form of schizophrenia, late paraphrenia and related disorders, for which specific medical treatment is available. Whatever the underlying cause of persecutory phenomena the health-care professionals' approach and ability to build workable relationships with a very difficult group of patients is cardinal to successful treatment.

REFERENCES

1. Howard, R.J., Forstl, H., Naguib, M. *et al.* (1992) First-rank symptoms of Schneider in late paraphrenia; cortical structural correlates. *British Journal of Psychiatry*, **160**, 108–9.
2. Cooper, A.F., Curry, A.R., Kay, D.W.K. *et al.* (1974) Hearing loss in paranoid and affective psychoses of the elderly. *Lancet*, **2**, 851–4.
3. Kalayman, B., Alexopoulos, G.S., Merrell, H.B. and Young, R.C. (1991) Patterns of hearing loss and psychiatric morbidity in elderly patients attending a hearing clinic. *International Journal of Geriatric Psychiatry*, **6**, 131–6.

4. Berrios, C.F. and Brook, P. (1984) Visual hallucinations and sensory delusions in the elderly. *British Journal of Psychiatry*, **144**, 662–4.
5. Quintal, M., Day-Cody, D. and Levy, R. (1991) Late paraphrenia and ICD10. *International Journal of Geriatric Psychiatry*, **6**, 111–16.
6. Roth, M. (1955) The natural history of mental disorder in old age. *Journal of Mental Science*, **101**, 281–301.
7. Grahame, P. (1982) Late paraphrenia. *British Journal of Hospital Medicine*, **27**, 522–8.
8. Post, F. (1971) Schizoaffective symptomatology in late life. *British Journal of Psychiatry*, **118**, 437–45.
9. Post, F. (1972) The management and nature of depressive illness in late life: a follow-through study. *British Journal of Psychiatry*, **121**, 393–404.
10. Roberts, G.W., Done, D.J., Bruton, C. and Crow, T.J. (1990) A 'mock up' of schizophrenia: temporal epilepsy and schizophrenia-like psychosis. *Biological Psychiatry*, **28**, 127–43.
11. Lemert, E.M. (1962) Paranoia and the dynamics of exclusion. *Sociometry*, **25**, 2–20.
12. Holden, U.P. and Woods, R.T. (1988) *Reality Orientation: Psychological Approaches to the 'Confused' Elderly*, 2nd edn, Churchill Livingstone, Edinburgh.

8

Psychological therapy with older people

No one remains free of problems or distress throughout their lives, but most people learn to cope with their problems or gain sufficient support and help from their personal relationships to overcome them. Some find that their distress becomes so great that their ability to cope with everyday life becomes seriously undermined. Elderly people have to face many changes specific to their age, as well as the range of problems that might occur at any time in life. Not only must they cope with changes in physical fitness and health, but they must also adapt to a wide variety of alterations, such as loss of earning power, attachments and status. Given this, most elderly people adapt well. It seems that it is the perception of younger people that the elderly are unhappy, rather than the complaint of old people themselves.

8.1 PSYCHOLOGICAL THERAPY

A simple way of conceptualizing psychological therapy is represented in Figure 8.1 which shows the interdependence between behaviour (actions), cognitions (beliefs and attitudes) and feelings or emotions in any situation. Psychological therapy aims at changing one or more elements of this triad, leaving the person better able to cope. The three groupings of therapeutic approaches for individuals which have some theoretical basis in psychology are the behaviour therapies, cognitive therapies and the psychodynamic therapies. In addition, there are techniques for understanding and helping groups, families and institutions.

Age is still seen by some as a contra-indication for psy-

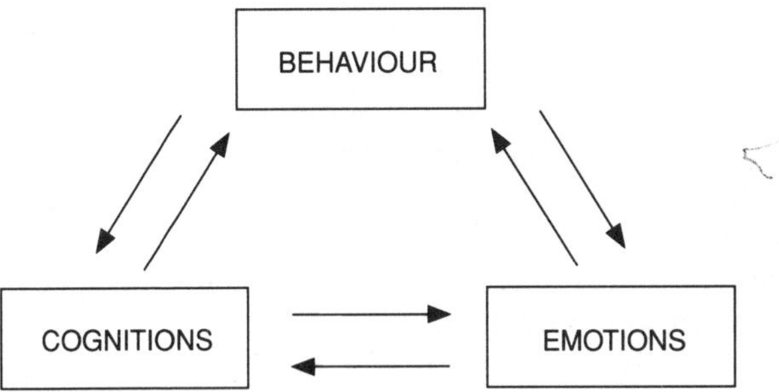

Figure 8.1 Psychological therapy: the interactive triad.

chological therapy, and still the majority of psychotherapeutic work is done with younger client groups. For those who have worked successfully with older patients, it is clear that it is quite possible to use the range of psychotherapeutic models in a conventional way, given some added knowledge of ageing. In terms of assessing an individual or family for a particular model, other salient criteria still need to be considered, but age in itself does not seem to preclude any approach. For example, whereas Freud himself expressed reservations about the use of psychoanalysis with older patients, there have been recent publications of case reports describing the successful analysis of patients in their seventies and eighties [1, 2]. Similar advances have been made in the use of behavioural approaches [3], cognitive therapies [4, 5], psychotherapy [6, 7], counselling [8] and family therapy [9]. In addition there are a number of approaches which have been developed specifically with old people in mind, such as Reality Orientation [10], Reminiscence [11] and Validation Therapy [12]. These are, in general, pragmatically based and derive their rationale from a variety of sources.

8.2 INDIVIDUAL PSYCHOLOGICAL APPROACHES

8.2.1 General issues

Individual psychological therapy can be considered when an individual is cognitively well-preserved, where the problem does not seem to be entirely defined by family members or carers and where the individual concerned both accepts that there is a problem and is willing to accept the role of psychological factors in the development and maintenance of problems rather than, for example, seeing them purely in physical terms. Individual therapy with elderly people requires all the skills and techniques which may be used with younger people, along with additional knowledge of the specific effects of ageing in the individual.

Whatever the therapeutic model and whatever the client's age, it is important in individual therapy to develop a therapeutic relationship, as this is necessary for co-operation in the use of therapeutic techniques, and may also produce change of itself [13]. This requires both an appropriate therapeutic attitude on the part of the professional and an informed client, whose expectations are realistic. All codes of therapeutic practice require that the therapist should show respect for the patient, refrain from exploiting or abusing patients, and accept the patient as a valued individual regardless of behaviour, thoughts or feelings. The therapist should listen, making active attempts to understand the problems that the patient is describing or displaying. There are techniques common to most therapies that help the patient to be open about emotional distress and to the therapist's interventions. These include reflecting back what the patient says and giving the patient an opportunity to correct the therapist. Genuineness, warmth and empathy are as important with older people as younger ones.

Some therapists are prepared to take the role of an active advocate for the patient. They justify this because age brings with it an increasing likelihood of physical infirmity and illness, so that it becomes harder to act on decisions or to take risks. Other therapists would not countenance this because to act on behalf of the patient outside therapy is to take a role inappropriate between two adults, and would be concerned to explore the difficulties described by the patient in, for example, mobilizing or accepting appropriate help, so that the patient herself may be enabled to pursue her goals. Either approach may be suitable, given a therapist of appropriate training, but it is necessary to be clear whether a particular approach suits the patient.

When the therapist is part of a multi-disciplinary team the

assistance of other members of the team in understanding and taking on extra-therapeutic tasks can be extremely helpful for the therapist attempting to maintain a particular role. For example, attendance at a day hospital may enable a patient to practise skills or extend themselves in a sheltered setting.

There is often a difficulty for the therapist in deciding on a setting. Reduced mobility often means that home visits or appointments during attendance for day hospital are required. Many practitioners feel that the initial assessment at least should always be conducted in the patient's home. In the end, a decision has to depend on circumstances and practicability. Sometimes the sheer physical obstacle of having to travel two or three miles to a hospital's outpatients' department may overcome the resources of the old person and outweigh their wish to receive therapeutic help; in other circumstances, it may only be possible to find an environment in which it is possible to think and work psychologically within a hospital setting. A home visit may increase the acceptability of therapy and the therapist can also get a clearer idea of how each individual copes in her own territory and can assess the degree to which social and environmental factors may be contributing to her difficulties. Those very factors, however, may inhibit therapy, if there is no opportunity for privacy, for example.

8.2.2 Therapeutic contracts

The overall process of therapy involves a number of stages, virtually regardless of approach or the characteristics of the patient (Figure 8.2). Following an assessment, therapist and patient come to an agreement about various aspects of the proposed therapy: they negotiate and agree a therapy contract. Sometimes the therapy contract is time-limited with a fixed number of sessions, or there is a set period followed by a review. It is important for patients to know of possible time limits, to allow them to regulate the strength of attachment towards the therapist, to pace themselves appropriately and to adjust to the ending of therapy. With old people, particular care must be taken in setting goals, the therapist holding in mind that someone in the latter part of their life may have priorities quite different from a younger person. Given also that ill or distressed old people can sometimes be reticent about

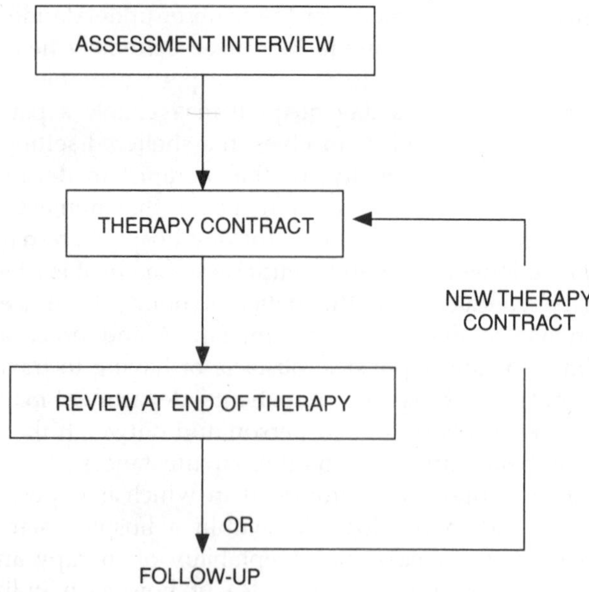

Figure 8.2 The therapy contract: a clear agreement is essential when working with elderly people.

asserting themselves, particularly against the wishes of those in authority, or in some circumstances are even not allowed to choose or decide for themselves, the therapist must be careful to ensure that therapeutic methods and goals are both realistic and desired by the patient.

8.2.3 Ageing, cognitive function and therapy

While it is clear that there are normal changes in cognitive abilities with increasing age, the practical impact of these is relatively minor. There are decreases in speed of information processing and reaction time, which may have important effects on success in complex tasks; expertise and skill may compensate for this. Older people tend to choose to respond accurately rather than rapidly. Old memories seem to be affected in the same way as more recent memories by age-related changes. Changes in intelligence seem to be variable. While some studies suggest a decrease in ability, others show a more mixed picture, with some individuals even increasing in intellectual ability as they reach old age. Major changes may well be [illegible] to organic conditions, such as Alzheimer's disease. High [illegible] improves memory performance, as does strategy [illegible] are no consistent age-related changes which influ[illegible]ty for therapy.

Bearing [illegible] mind, there are some changes in cognitive function whi[illegible] commonly encountered and which may have direct implications for therapy with some individuals [15]. Such changes in ability may cause difficulties when the therapist fails to use language, concepts or imagery familiar to the client, but uses technical language or jargon. The over-65 population is not homogeneous, there being statistically a difference between young elderly and very old people. This reaffirms the importance of assessing the individual elderly person's needs and assets before carrying out a therapeutic intervention. However, in spite of the reality of these changes, it is likely that emotional and social factors will be a more important part in most cases where cognitive impairment is not at issue.

It is important with older, as with younger people, to be aware of the effect of presenting unfamiliar or large amounts of information in circumstances which might hinder its retention. Time limits require thought on the therapist's part and some therapists advocate a more structured approach, with an emphasis on concrete and practical issues, generous time limits and even written instructions. Research has shown that the average young person will forget at least one-half of the verbal instructions given by a GP within five minutes of leaving the surgery. Ley [16] has made several specific suggestions for increasing the amount of information patients are likely to recall, which may be useful (see Table 8.1).

Table 8.2 offers a summary of factors which should be considered. These may not always be necessary or appropriate, but may make all the difference to outcome in some cases. A psychological approach will often need to be co-ordinated with appropriate medical and social interventions and this may influence what change is possible.

Elderly people do not necessarily find it more difficult to accept help from a younger person, but there is perhaps a danger that a younger therapist will find it harder to under-

Table 8.1 Suggestions for increasing amount and content of patients' recall

1. Whenever possible, provide patients with instructions and advice at the start of the information to be presented
2. When providing patients with instructions and advice, stress how important they are
3. Use short words and short sentences
4. Use explicit categorization where possible
5. Repeat things where feasible
6. When giving advice make it as specific, detailed and concrete as possible

Table 8.2 Factors enhancing therapeutic contact with elderly people

1. Less abstract, interpretative approach
2. Compensate for reduction in memory for meaning
3. Flexible session length (client comfort)
4. Flexibility of session location (client's home versus office)
5. Time-limited contract
6. Explicit, concrete, realistic goals
7. Awareness of real social and physical limitations
8. Provision of formal social resources and support
9. Awareness of the interpersonal context of problem ('family' or 'institutional')
10. Active rather than passive therapist
11. Awareness of age contrast in goal-setting and empathy
12. Awareness of ageism in therapist
13. Awareness of drug effects in the elderly
14. Assessment of physical factors which may exacerbate psychological problems

stand the priorities of and constraints on an older person. Just as there has been an interest in the experience of women, since it is clear that women are neither like men nor their opposites, so it is the case that older people are neither like younger ones nor do they necessarily fit the stereotypes offered to us. Nor are old people a homogeneous group. Education, class and gender may affect both the old person's attitudes and our expectations, in addition to personal style, physical status and age itself. The age span described as elderly in our society covers around 35 years, enough to contain three generations. There are still prejudices about old people, and to some extent

Table 8.5 Mr G.S.'s problems and treatment methods

Problem	*Therapeutic approach*	*Therapy involves*
Illegal sexual behaviour and related fantasy and dreaming	Covert sensitization	Associating images of illegal sexual behaviour with highly unpleasant consequences
No sexual response to adult females	Orgasmic reconditioning	Associating stimulation and ejaculation with conventional fantasy
No constructive life Lots of free time	Support and problem-solving	Looking at and encouraging possible interests
Anger and shame related to previous events	Empathy and re-evaluation of events	Allowing expression of feelings and helping to re-evaluate them

Case history 8.3:

Mrs H.S. was referred with feelings of depression some time after the death of her husband. She felt she had not come to terms with his death and that she could not make a life of her own. It became clear over a period of time that Mrs H.S. had in fact never really had a life of her own. First, she had looked after her mother, who was widowed, then she had married and brought up children. Her husband had always lived an independent life, working hard for the family but rarely having much free time at home. There was a clear indication that he had not wanted his wife to work or to go out much without him, and Mrs H.S. had gone along with this to keep the peace. After first her mother then her husband died, Mrs H.S. felt both guilty and anxious about asserting herself. She even felt that she might not deserve therapy, as there must be others who needed it more. This led to anger about all the restrictions on her life, directed both at her loved ones and at herself. When these issues were discussed openly, Mrs H.S. began to consider her options and made arrangements to go on holiday with a friend and to join social activities. When, some time later, a friend proposed marriage, she refused, saying that she was enjoying herself too much and did not want to give up her hard-won independence. Termination involved consideration of Mrs H.S.'s future, her sadness at yet another loss (that of the therapist) and a sense of achievement. At one year follow-up Mrs H.S. remained well.

8.2.5 Common client issues

Developmental models all share the premise that growth occurs through the resolution of conflict. Ageing brings with it changes in attitudes, health and looks which affect self-image and relationships, alteration in status at work with either increased experience or competition with younger colleagues, generational changes as parents die and children mature, changes in sexual functioning and marital relationships, and an awareness of time and mortality. These themes all appear regularly in clinical work with old people as they face the realities of retirement or illness, and, as stated earlier, much therapeutic work with older people involves facing and coming to terms with losses of several types. There is the most commonly understood loss, of a person or relationship, commonly experienced in old age as peers die. There are also losses experienced as a result of social change, such as the loss of status, occupation, power and money through retirement. There are also other types of loss, most notably physical (loss of health, looks or mobility, for example) or psychological (e.g. loss of a view of oneself as potent or of a belief such as, 'It will never happen to me').

There are several models of the process of mourning and of bereavement counselling [19]. Most recognize stages of taking in the fact of the loss, protest or attempts to undo the loss, despair or active mourning, then a phase of reinvesting in new people or activities. The stages are not clearly defined; rather it is more that the loss is recognized anew many times and has to be mourned again and again. It is when this process goes wrong or becomes stuck in some way that people sometimes become patients. This might occur when the fact of the loss is not accepted or is denied (e.g. the man who remarries immediately his wife dies), or if the person remains out of touch with her feelings (e.g. the one who stays calm in order to hold things together when everyone else is too upset), or if she remains in a stage of despair (e.g. the woman who feels useless and worthless once she feels her good looks are gone or her role as a maternal figure is over). Difficulties may be exacerbated if the person who dies is idealized, or if the patient feels both hostility and guilt towards the deceased.

What is less clear is that there are compensations which come with age for many people, who may mourn what is lost, but can make something worthwhile from the resources and opportunities available to them. The therapist should consider the options available to a patient and consider whether this patient is able to use these, and what change is necessary to facilitate the best use of resources. It may be a lack of self-esteem that prevents a widow from attending local activities and making new contacts; her depressed mood may be due less to unresolved grief than anxiety over starting over again. While she may well miss her husband, it might be that his function for her as a constant companion reduced the necessity to overcome long-standing feelings of social anxiety or difficulties in asserting herself. Such an individual may present with somatic symptoms, depressed mood or anxiety. Where a difficulty in coming to accept a loss is the issue, it may be that the patient is avoiding pain for what she feels is good reason, perhaps because she believes she will not be able to survive the feelings of loss. The task of the therapist is both to provide a benign, containing environment in which the patient may feel it is safe to express her feelings about the loss, and to help her recognize that avoidance of those feelings blocks the mourning process.

Case history 8.4:

Mrs F.S. was a 66-year-old woman who gradually developed a depressive illness including marked obsessional checking behaviour. As she responded to anti-depressant medication the community nurse involved requested psychological advice about her obsessional behaviour.

Assessment identified a further problem, that of an unresolved bereavement reaction regarding the death of her husband four years previously. A programme aimed at treating the obsessional behaviour and sessions of bereavement counselling were apparently successfully completed by the community nurse. Since the community nurse was leaving to obtain further training, the clinical psychologist agreed to carry out a follow-up. At one month follow-up it was found that Mrs F.S. was experiencing 'panics' once or twice weekly within the home and an anxiety-management plan was instituted. However, it soon became apparent that she was becoming depressed again (the anti-depressants had been discontinued). Although she initially denied there was anything to make her depressed, careful questioning elicited the fact that she regularly had thoughts about her dead husband, but tended to push them out of her mind because they upset her. She also found it impossible to get out a picture of her husband, which she had put away because it upset her. Clearly, despite the community nurse's efforts, her bereavement was still unresolved. It was agreed with the GP to re-institute anti-depressant medication to prevent her from becoming more depressed and a series of bereavement-treatment sessions was instituted. It was found in this case that just talking about the husband and his death did not necessarily elicit any apparent upset or emotion. It was only through the use of specific objects she was avoiding, such as the husband's photograph and by asking her to visualize disturbing personal scenes, such as her husband dying in her arms, that she was able to experience the distressing emotions of bereavement. Using this approach, the emotions gradually lessened and although the sessions themselves were extremely stressful for both herself and the therapist, she was always able to experience a feeling of relief by the end of the session.

Case history 8.5:

Mrs D.G. had found that her husband, who suffered from Alzheimer's disease, was too impaired for her to look after, and she agreed to his admission to a Residential Home. Some weeks later, she became very distressed, when, as is often the case, the staff informed her that her husband was no bother to look after. This made Mrs D.G. feel guilty. She was also feeling lonely without him, it being too early for her to have established other social routines. Over a number of sessions Mrs D.G. talked over her feelings about her loss, the conflict she felt over seeing her husband in the Home and her attempts to make a new life for herself. At six months, she felt she was getting back on her feet and agreed to a follow-up appointment in six months, at which point she felt able to be discharged.

Not only do old people have to deal with the death of others, but they have to face the prospect of their own death. One survey of healthy elderly people found that while 55 per cent showed a realistic judgement or resolution to death, 30 per cent showed overt fear and 15 per cent denial [20]. Fear of death may need to be understood in the context of the person's life, and may comprise a number of anxieties, such as fear of pain, loss of self or loneliness, or may result from feelings that life has been too short or unfair. Although techniques such as systematic desensitization and thought-stopping have been suggested to reduce fear of death in elderly clients, there is no evidence as to their effectiveness. Counselling and psychotherapeutic approaches have more to offer. For some, the chance to request factual information may be a relief. For others it may be helpful to find that they are constructing a fearful idea of dying, based on past experiences, but still an idea not a fact. Some use their religion to offer comfort.

The five cases presented illustrate a variety of approaches to psychological problems in intellectually intact old people based on a logical appraisal of problems and the use of appropriate techniques, some specialized and some relatively simple, to tackle problems.

8.3 FAMILY THERAPY

The well-being of the older person is affected by those around her. Many elderly people live either with a spouse or other relative and even those who live alone often have some contact with relatives who are within easy travelling distance. With many elderly people, the understanding of the family context may be the key to finding the most appropriate psychological approach. Changes such as retirement, illness and bereavement alter patterns of dependency and activity within the family. Increasingly, family therapy is being seen as a valuable and effective method for families in which there are difficulties in adapting to transitions due to ageing [21, 22].

Rather than providing a particular conceptual model of family therapy, the aim in this section is to alert readers to the potential for family therapy with elderly people and their families and the use of some commonly used concepts.

8.3.1 The interactional system

The focus of assessment is the family system and the interactions of its different members. Thus the involvement of the other members of the family in perpetuating the distressed or disturbing behaviour of the elderly referred patient is emphasized. This can be illustrated by considering a family in which the father and mother lived together and their only daughter visited regularly.

Case history 8.6:

Before Mr P.K.'s retirement, the family felt there were no problems. He worked, his wife was a conscientious housewife and their daughter visited every day to spend time with her. All were used to their particular roles and related to each other in ways which promoted mutual psychological well-being. However, on Mr P.K.'s retirement, he found he had little with which to occupy his time. He tried to transfer his skills for organizing to the home and began to take over long-established routines and household tasks, thus usurping a role which his wife had seen as her own. It seemed that Mrs P.K. felt that she may have gained a husband, but she lost her privacy, her autonomy and her exclusive time with her daughter. This led to heated arguments between husband and wife. Their daughter, who saw this as interference by her father, sided with her mother. Thus Mr P.K., who had lost the status and self-esteem he had at work, was now also faced with antagonism from his daughter and wife, and lapsed into helpless depression and hostility. The system was balanced in a new way, dependent on his 'illness'. Treating Mr P.K.'s depression with medication was not sufficient to make him well. The family system had to be explored and altered so that he had a role which did not antagonize his wife and yet enabled him to regain his self-esteem.

8.3.2 Faulty problem-solving

Most family members are caring and attempt to help the referred person, even when these family members appear difficult, intransigent or, occasionally, openly destructive. In general, the family members have attempted to solve problems which have arisen from a change in life circumstance in one or more family members. It is when these attempts at problem-solving are faulty that the initial problems can be exacerbated, leading eventually to the elderly family member being referred for psychiatric help.

In the previous example, it can be seen that initially the father made an attempt to solve his own problems, i.e. finding a new role which would maintain his self-esteem and use up the extra eight hours in the day. What he did not take into account was the combined resentment that resulted from his competition for the role of organizer in the home. His daughter's response to this was also an attempt to solve a problem, that of the arguments between her father and mother, by supporting her mother to resist change. This placed the problem back with Mr P.K. and he, rather than try an alternative activity, became depressed.

8.3.3 Setting the scene for family therapy

The initial contact between therapist and family and how this is organized is an important factor in making interventions successful. Two guidelines may be helpful in communicating to the family members that the team see the problem as one for the whole family, rather than an issue for the referred patient alone. Some patients may be referred for family work during an admission to hospital. In these circumstances, it may be better to wait and see the whole family together after discharge. Second, copies of the appointment letter need to be sent to all invited members of the family individually, including the referred patient. This may state that the therapists are aware that the problem affects the whole family and that all family members have a part to play, thus placing the responsibility squarely on the family rather than just on one person.

8.3.4 Information-gathering

It is beneficial, especially where the therapists are less experienced in working with families, that at least two professionals work together. This has a number of advantages. Large amounts of information coming from a variety of different family members can be difficult for one therapist to follow effectively. If both sexes are represented on the co-therapist's team, they may get much more information from the family. A further problem in carrying out family therapy can be the powerful way in which family members present their view of the situation. For example, they may see the patient as mentally ill, and that the problem is for her to change or for the therapists to return her to her previous condition. Two therapists are more likely to meet such situations constructively.

As in all psychological therapy the gathering of information from a number of sources is important. Where a member of the family has been an inpatient, staff reports of the interactions between the relatives and the patient can provide useful information about how the family works, while the GP, through his contact and longer-term knowledge of the family, can provide invaluable background information.

In initial interview sessions with the whole family present, therapists are interested not only in what is being said and how it is said, but also in the non-verbal communication within the family. The next case history illustrates a feature of particular relevance to ageing, as in a subsequent session it became clear that the patient's sister-in-law felt that the patient herself could not have a valid point of view because her illness must mean that she was senile.

Case history 8.7:

This family consisted of two sisters aged 70 and 71 living together. One, who had been admitted to hospital when she was mute and unco-operative, had just been discharged. The other sister was due to be discharged from hospital following a cataract operation. Both sisters were visited regularly by their brother and sister-in-law. The initial session involved the sister who had just been discharged, her brother and sister-in-law. The sister-in-law sat next to the sister clutching at the sister's dress and patting her knee as if she were a child, while stridently talking across her to the therapist. The brother complained the sister was as ill as ever and still mute. When the therapist insisted that the sister-in-law address her questions to the 'mute' sister she protested vigorously and had to be repeatedly directed to do this. Even when she did direct a question to her sister, she never waited for a reply, often answering the question herself as soon as she had asked it! Interestingly, her husband had a pronounced stammer and even he had difficulty getting a word in edgeways. By the end of the session the 'mute' sister had begun to talk and, although this was only the beginning of a complicated family-therapy case, a great deal of information had been gathered.

A case of a mother and daughter living together illustrates two important aspects of communication in a family therapy.

Case history 8.8:

Following a referral from her GP, Mrs M.M., a 70-year-old widow, was admitted with a possible depressive illness. While on the ward, she was started on anti-depressant medication, although the severity of her depression was in some doubt. On her discharge, her daughter, Ms B.M., expressed considerable concern about how her mother would cope. Shortly afterwards, the daughter made 'desperate' contact with her two GPs and the ward staff, eventually bringing her mother back two days early to see 'anybody'. The daughter's response was out of all proportion to what was known of the mother's state. The conflicting advice Ms B.M. was managing to get from different members of the team effectively prevented the assigned therapists from making any progress. The situation only improved after a team meeting (a rather heated one!) in which the therapists reached an agreement with other members of the team that the daughter should be channelled in their direction. As therapy progressed, it became clear that the mother's depression was a reaction to her daughter's bouts of excessive drinking and disastrous adventures with men. A vicious downward spiral of her daughter's drinking worsening the mother's depression and criticism of her daughter, leading to more drinking by the daughter, was interrupted by a series of therapeutic interventions. One of these involved the therapists communicating their view of the positive aspects of the apparently destructive behaviour of each woman and expressing their belief in the strength of the attachment of both. This family dyad remained vulnerable as neither had, nor facilitated the other to have, outside interests or social contacts, but the drinking bouts reduced and Mrs M.M. has not been readmitted.

This case illustrates the problems that can arise when a number of different professionals and agencies are working with a family. GPs and social workers are often the most vulnerable in this respect and it is important, when they know some family work is being done, that they listen sympathetically, but do not feel obliged to give advice beyond asking the family to contact their therapist. This may also occur with individuals and is a common difficulty when working with older people because so often there are a number of professionals and agencies involved.

Another important aspect of communication in family therapy is how the therapists communicate to the family members the ways in which they might need to change. There are several techniques in comon usage, such as positive connotation, in which the efforts of family members are recognized and valued. This disarms the person concerned, who may be anxious that she will be criticized. Recognition that a behaviour is an attempt to solve the problem is more helpful than criticism and is more likely to lead on to change in the behaviour. One way of acknowledging the efforts the family have made is to assess in detail what solutions the family (and other agencies) have tried and failed. This also provides the therapist with clues about what solutions may help the family, and allows the therapist to assess how well previous solutions have been implemented. Circular questioning is another strategy which allows all family members to offer their opinions, and this proved valuable in both cases described above. This involves asking the members of the family their view of a situation, often of another member's opinion or feelings.

It is important when using family-therapy techniques to consider the impact of transitions for the family member concerned and, in addition, the impact of these on other members as sometimes the needs of one may come into conflict with the responsibilities of others. For example, the wish for a 69-year-old widow to have her 34-year-old daughter stay closely involved while she comes to terms with the death of her husband, may be felt to interfere with the daughter's need to consolidate a relationship in which she can have children.

8.4 BEHAVIOURAL PROBLEMS

There are many possible factors contributing to a behaviour, some of which may be environmental, others internal to the person. Behaviours may be affected by near factors, such as the immediate behaviour of other people, or by distant factors, such as social change. Most of the time people understand and manage their own and other people's behaviours as well as they need, but sometimes a person may behave in ways that are troubling or dangerous to themselves or others. This kind of referral is commonly made to services for old people. The referred patient may or may not be suffering from dementia. Often the behaviour is felt by others to be at least partially under the voluntary control of the patient. This leads to difficulty if reasoning with the patient has no effect on the behaviour. Troubling behaviours include aggression, inappropriate sexual activities, dangerous behaviours, rejection of care or control, and stereotyped or repetitive behaviour (see

Table 8.6 Common troubling behaviours

1. Hostile and aggressive behaviours, including threats, verbal abuse and physical violence to self or others
2. Dangerous and risky behaviours, including wandering, leaving on gas taps, self-neglect
3. Socially inappropriate behaviours, including some sexual interactions, disinhibition, bad manners, sloppy eating or incontinence
4. Excessive demands for care and attention
5. Stereotyped behaviours and repetitive requests
6. Withdrawal, passivity, apathy
7. Rejection of help, and unreasonable conditions for accepting help

Table 8.6). Sleeplessness and incontinence are also commonly reported problems.

Sometimes the referrer describes the behaviour as attention-seeking, although such behaviours are not always aimed to gain attention. The risk of a description like this is that it provides little information, and can lead to a person being dismissed or treated in a denigrating way, provoking more distressed behaviour. The authors have heard the label 'confused', for example, used to describe not only someone who could not find the way around a ward or to the toilet, but also someone who did not accept that she was in hospital, and someone who tried to 'escape' regularly from a Home to see her (long dead) husband. Only a detailed description of the problem behaviour and circumstances surrounding it can allow the development of a constructive management plan.

A behavioural assessment will involve observation and measurement of behaviour. These approaches are often quantitative in nature. In addition, the aim of assessment may be to clarify sequences of events in order to identify triggers and consequences of a particular behaviour. The function of the behaviour for the patient and others can then be better understood. This model is illustrated in Figure 8.3. The return arrow shows that sometimes the consequences of a behaviour may contribute to its repetition, even leading to a vicious circle.

The procedure may be as follows: a baseline measurement of the behaviour is taken, for example, information on the number of times a patient is incontinent in a week, which allows the psychologist to measure the extent of a problem and

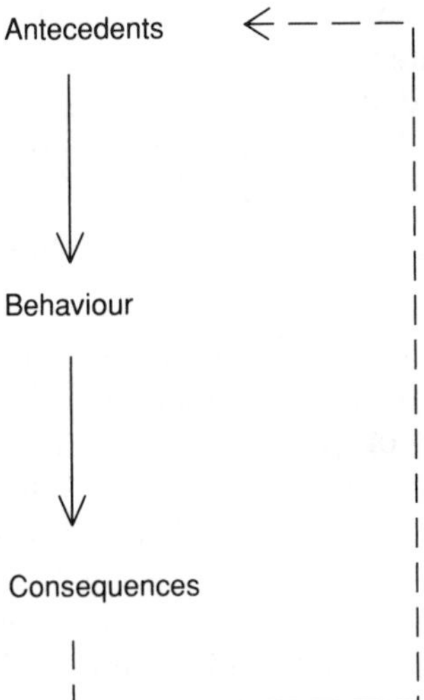

Figure 8.3 Antecedents, behaviour, consequences.

then measure the effects of a treatment. This is easiest with discrete symptoms or easily defined behaviours. If the frequency is fairly stable, say, twice a day most days, the planned intervention might then be put into action. If there is no pattern, so that the patient is incontinent several times a day in the first few days, then not at all for the last few, it is preferable to collect more information. The frequency of incontinence can then be measured either consistently throughout the period of the intervention or at intervals. Ratings should be continued through each intervention and for a period afterwards, so that the effects of the treatment itself and of stopping the treatment can be seen. Case history 8.9 illustrates the use of a simple assessment procedure and behavioural regime for helping a patient minimize incontinence.

Case history 8.9:

Mrs G.J. was referred with incontinence. Staff were asked to keep a record of the number of times each day that she suffered from this. After two weeks, they had produced a diary. It was agreed that Mrs G.J. might benefit from following a regular toiletting regime. Mrs G.J. became ill with a chest infection and the regime was stopped and not reintroduced until several weeks after her recovery. As Mrs G.J. did not remember to go to the bathroom herself, and the benefits were clear, the staff decided to keep up the regular reminders, but stopped recording.

A careful analysis of behaviour will often facilitate the development of appropriate formulation and treatment. Table 8.7 describes a range of possible causes and strategies for incontinence to show the variety of possible approaches to consider in any one problem. This shows how analysing a behaviour can involve the consideration of many factors and also that some analyses of behaviour problems may not lead to behavioural interventions. Publications which focus on the

Table 8.7 Urinary incontinence in a confused person

Reason	*Strategy*
1. Medical (e.g. urinary tract infection)	Treat medical condition
2. Incontinence being reinforced	Reward periods of dryness, e.g. by staff attention
3. Cannot find toilet (short-term memory impairment)	Practice, use of a variety of cues, and signposting
4. Cannot recognize toilet (visual agnosia)	Use a colour code, e.g. only red in unit is toilet doors
5. Cannot get to toilet in time (mobility)	Increase accessibility of toilet
6. Stress incontinence	Pelvic floor muscle exercises
7. Cannot dress or undress	Practise dressing/undressing skills
8. Toilet uncomfortable (e.g. commode seat-top missing)	Make more comfortable
9. Lack of motivation	Encourage and reinforce successful toileting and dryness
10. Cannot understand verbal instructions to find toilet (receptive aphasia)	Use alternative cue, e.g. visual
11. Cannot express need for toilet (expressive aphasia)	Sensitize staff to individual's attempt to communicate needs. Knowledge of individual's routine

management of specific problems include a series of books by Graham Stokes [23, 24, 25, 26] concerned with the assessment and management of incontinence and other difficulties. The principles of sleep hygiene are outlined in a volume by Morgan and Gledhill (27). With a co-operative patient or a behaviour in which medical or social factors play the major part, simple behavioural programmes or modifications to institutional practice and living arrangements may have a significant effect.

In the following case history, a simple analysis led to a solution involving more than one strategy. It also illustrates how, often, a problem behaviour comes about if the old person is unable to communicate their needs, or their strategy to gain satisfaction of ordinary human needs is unacceptable to others. Sometimes a problem behaviour comes about as a way of dealing with anxiety. The problem behaviour may be the best possible solution available to the old person without help. A successful intervention is likely to be one which takes into account the meaning and function of the behaviour, and enables a patient's needs to be satisfied in a mutually satisfactory way.

Case history 8.10:

Mrs A.O., who was suffering from dementia, was referred by the staff of the Residential Home in which she lived because she was continually shouting. On observing the situation, it quickly became clear that she was shouting out names. The other residents ignored Mrs A.O. or occasionally shouted back at her, and she seemed isolated. The staff thought she was calling them, but the psychologist noticed that the shouts became worse after one of her daughters visited. The daughter was able to confirm that the names her mother called had belonged to her sisters, who were now either dead or infirm and unable to visit. The psychologist felt that Mrs A.O. was lonely and that her shouts had resulted, not in the company she had wanted, but a rejection by the other residents. She asked the staff to make contact with Mrs A.O. on a regular basis, by just chatting to her as they passed by. She also offered to spend some time helping the staff to set up and run a Reminiscence group, of which Mrs A.O. became a member. With established contact, first from staff, then residents, Mrs A.O.'s need to shout decreased, resulting in permanent improvement.

Sometimes, a simple behavioural analysis is enough. When those involved in the situation are distressed or if the behaviour is dangerous, a more complex analysis may be necessary. Then, clarifying the meaning of the behaviour for both the referred patient and others is important. For example, in some Residential Homes, where the staff are used to high levels of incontinence or asocial behaviour, a person exhibiting such problems may be happily tolerated, while in another, the behaviour may be considered unacceptable and lead to the person being rejected by fellow residents or staff, or even being required to move. Further, while carers can often understand and cope well with incontinence *per se*, deliberate soiling is often experienced as extremely distressing. Sometimes, strategies which are intended to deal with a problem can exacerbate it. The staff caring for Mrs A.O., for example, thought they were right to ignore her shouts, because that would only encourage her in the behaviour. Without the Reminiscence group, this might have been the case, but the psychologist could see beyond the nuisance value of the shouting and was able to envisage an alternative strategy that allowed for the satisfaction of Mrs A.O.'s needs by her peers. This case illustrates well the need for careful consideration of the old person's well-being.

Common psychological functions of troubling behaviours may include the avoidance of isolation, the maintenance of either control or self-esteem, or the expression of feelings through action rather than words. Such functions need to be considered in addition to the more accepted features of organic impairment such as a reduced capacity to inhibit acting upon impulses or a decreased ability to employ abstract thought processes. In addition, it is useful, when making such an assessment, to know of past patterns of behaviour when under stress. For example, some individuals have habitually resorted to physical violence when frustrated; others may feel ill or demand help. Long-standing strategies imply that the individual has been strongly reinforced for this behaviour and may well have developed a set of attitudes which support its use. Such behaviours may be hard to modify.

Behavioural approaches often require the co-operation and active participation of relatives and staff and, whenever possible, the patient. Occasionally, it may need an amount of diplomacy to explain an analysis of some problems to the staff or relatives involved, especially if their reaction serves to exacerbate the problem. It is also important to consider the constraints under which relatives or staff may have to operate. Examples of such constraints include fatigue and limitations of physical strength, environmental design and the concern for the safety of the patient themselves and other people in the vicinity of the patient, the effects on quality of life for the patient and others, and finally, ethical and legal considerations.

Case history 8.11:

Mrs N.M. was referred by ward staff because she shouted for help, but when asked what she wanted she could not say. She could sometimes be verbally abusive. When she was assessed it appeared that the behaviour was limited to particular times in the day and to one or two settings on the ward. Mrs N.M. would shout at fairly regular intervals if left on her own or in a group of patients, but the frequency of shouts increased when a staff member walked by. This had been going on for some time: Mrs N.M. was at the end of a protracted period of assessment, and it was felt that the shouting was the main problem left, holding up discharge to a nursing home. Mrs N.M. was mildly cognitively impaired, but her relatives lived too far away to help her at home. The staff had already tried to ignore the shouts, in the hope that extinction would occur. However, Mrs N.M. had become increasingly distressed and agitated, eventually ending in an incident in which she had pushed another patient. The staff were anxious that someone would be hurt. At the time of the assessment, some staff were tolerant of the shouts, and spoke warmly to Mrs N.M. Others were frustrated by the difficulty of resolving the problem, so that Mrs N.M. would sometimes be asked to wait or told not to shout. On a number of occasions, after being scolded, Mrs N.M. apologized, after which the staff member concerned would feel guilty and Mrs N.M. would end up getting a hug. This seemed mutually very satisfying, but it was clear that the staff response to Mrs N.M. maintained the problem behaviour. It was possible to implement two strategies in this case. The interval between shouts was averaged at about ten minutes, so members of staff were initially asked to speak to Mrs N.M. when she was in the day room or the quiet room about every eight minutes, if she was not shouting at the time. This did not always have to be a conversation but could just be a word or two in passing. Staff wondered if Mrs N.M. was needing this contact because she was upset about leaving her own home and anxious about her future and one nurse was allocated to talk over possible options and anxieties with Mrs N.M. She was prepared to go over the same discussion several times until Mrs N.M. was reassured. This was followed by a series of visits to a nursing home, and eventually Mrs N.M. was happily transferred.

Here it was possible to successfully change a situation in which the staff and patient's behaviours were being maintained by the other. Other factors which had an effect were the behaviour of other patients (sometimes difficult to change), emotional, social and medical factors and life circumstances. Designing a successful intervention may require ingenuity. It may be possible to change the behaviour of the referred patient; sometimes it may be necessary for others in the environment to change in order to achieve this. Sometimes, the characteristics of the behaviour or limits in the home or institutional setting may make change difficult to achieve.

One difficulty is the tendency to see disturbing behaviour in others as symptomatic of illness on the one hand, or as deliberately antisocial on the other. While both illness and choice over behaviour may be important, it is often only a detailed assessment that shows up how different factors may interact and suggests possible foci. A further element to take into account is the impact of disturbing behaviour on those around. This may well mean that carers and peers are impaired in their ability to cope through the feelings aroused in them by the behaviour. They may react under stress in ways that exacerbate the problem. Often within institutions and families, feelings may run high, leading to avoidance, guilt, punitive behaviour or scapegoating. Sometimes, one of the tasks of assessment is to estimate how possible it is for the others in the situation to change too. After all, especially when the patient is cognitively impaired, it may be only the carers who have the capacity to consistently effect any change. It is sometimes possible to understand more about the functions of a behaviour for a patient by thinking about the feelings aroused in others. For example, attempts to control others, whether through aggressive attack or attention-seeking, may arouse feelings of fear, impotence or anger as well as more sympathetic responses. This may be a clue to the difficulty experienced by the patient, who may resort to disturbing behaviours to cope with overwhelming or uncomprehended feelings of fear, for example, of isolation, anger or helplessness.

The following case suggests the limits on what can be achieved. Staff in this situation were sufficiently concerned about the safety of other residents to remove Mr A.V.'s electric wheelchair. As this was essential for independent mobility, Mr A.V. felt he had been punished and this led to increased hostility. A long-standing pattern of aggressive behaviour in response to frustration or constraint proved difficult to modify.

Case history 8.12:

Mr A.V. was referred by staff within the Residential Home in which he lived. Over a period of three months, he had been sexually harassing female residents. Although he had been seen by staff members, he had denied any such activity. Mr A.V. was confined to an electric wheelchair and, when the incidents did not stop, the staff removed this so that Mr A.V. was immobilized. He became violent towards staff, hitting them when they came to help him transfer. At this point, help was requested. It was clear that Mr A.V. had become resentful of what he felt was a punishment, but it was more difficult to understand why the sexual assaults had started in the first place. In the meantime, both staff and residents were understandably anxious about restoring Mr A.V.'s wheelchair and the possibility of further incidents, while Mr A.V. was unwilling to co-operate with anyone, even refusing to talk. After some enquiry, it was found that Mr A.V.'s wife, who had suffered physical violence for much of her married life, had decided that she had taken enough, and after having arranged his admission and ensured its permanence, had decided she no longer wished to visit her husband. Mr A.V. was therefore reduced to expressing his rage with her on the female residents and staff. In this case, the initial input was limited to advice on management and avoidance of the violence. It was possible to limit Mr A.V.'s care to male or mixed-sex pairs of staff. Firm but understanding management allowed for the problem to be contained over a period of months and it became possible to converse with Mr A.V. in a friendly manner. However, he never really came to accept or mourn the loss of his wife, nor did staff feel that other residents would necessarily be safe with Mr A.V. back in his electric wheelchair. Eventually, he died from a second stroke.

Behavioural assessment attempts to clarify the relationship between the environment and the behaviour of the patient. However, any behaviour may be affected by a number of factors. A primary dysfunction may subsequently be affected by secondary handicap and then by what has been termed opportunistic handicap [28]. The last example illustrates this.

Case history 8.13:

Mr S.C. was referred by his GP who was worried about the effects of his behaviour on his wife. Dr Smith felt that if the situation did not improve Mrs S.C. would no longer be able to cope with caring for him, and that he would have to go into a Residential Home. Mr S.C. suffered from minor memory and language difficulties following a stroke. He had lost his mother at nine years old and had spent the remainder of his childhood living with an aunt, who was remembered by his wife as critical and distant.

He married in his twenties and became the dominant partner, wanting to control his wife's routine and limit her outside activities and friendships. The couple had one daughter, who left home in her teens because she felt her father restricted her. On marriage, she moved away and had little contact with her parents. Mr S.C. hated being dependent on his wife, attempting to restrict her from leaving the house. Often, he refused to help himself by dressing or using the lavatory appropriately although he was capable of doing these independently, albeit slowly. On these occasions, he seemed to enjoy the distress of his wife, which possibly allowed him to feel powerful and in control even if at the cost of a good relationship with her. Problematic behaviour became noticeably worse if his wife made any arrangement that did not suit him. He refused to think about or to plan for his future needs with his wife or the doctor, and would become hostile if anyone tried to discuss his disability, refusing to accept the loss of his once physically healthy self. In this instance, Mrs S.C. was given counselling to help her work out ways of coping with her husband with only moderate success.

8.5 SPECIALIZED THERAPEUTIC APPROACHES

A number of approaches have been developed with the needs of old people in mind. These include Reality Orientation [10], Reminiscence [11] and Validation Therapy [12]. A short explanation of each is outlined below, but there are references for the reader interested in pursuing these at the end of the chapter.

8.5.1 Reality Orientation

This was first introduced into this country from the United States, where it was developed as a method of orientating individuals who were suffering from memory impairment, especially dementia, to the details of their environment. Reality Orientation comes in two forms. In the 24-hour or informal approach, the emphasis is on aiding the person within their environment. Members of staff would repetitively provide relevant information on time, place, person and routine, for example. Also, the environment itself can be modified by the use of signs in several modes (such as the written word plus a picture), colour coding calendars and equipment such as outsize clocks. This aimed primarily at making up for the individual's memory loss at a specific time, but it was also hoped that the information would be retained. This informal approach was reinforced by group or classroom sessions which served to provide information and stimulation of varying types. In practice, this can range from basic information on names and dates, through current affairs, sensory input and reminiscence. In addition to any improvement in retention of factual information, it is clear that these groups can serve a valuable function as a social setting in which individuals suffering from a cognitive impairment can become involved in conversation with others, both patients and staff. There can be improvements in mood and self-esteem for the group members, while staff often report that they can learn more about patients in a group setting.

8.5.2 Life Review and Reminiscence

Life Review [29] is an approach based on psychotherapeutic principles. It is assumed that individuals may benefit from an opportunity to reconsider their lives. The remembering and re-evaluation of past decisions and trauma with a skilled therapist to contain feelings of, for example, distress or grief, will allow the more realistic appraisal of current conflicts, problems and opportunities. It is considered appropriate for people suffering from emotional distress rather than an organic disorder.

Reminiscence, on the other hand, aims to increase self-esteem through sharing memories of past events with peers and a group leader. There are both informal and structured approaches, and, as is the case with Reality Orientation, there is a range of standard materials offered for sale. With this kind of concrete material provided, it is possible to use Reminiscence with a wide range of patients, including those with dementia.

8.5.3 Validation Therapy

The practice of Validation Therapy [12] requires the staff member to attempt to understand the feelings behind a behaviour or communication and to affirm these, rather than focus on possibly erroneous factual details communicated by a patient suffering from a memory or language difficulty. As such, it is useful as a way of responding to behaviours and communications of patients who are unable to express their needs or emotions because of cognitive impairment.

Apart from Life Review, these therapeutic approaches are designed for, or are primarily used with people suffering from dementia, and as such represent an attempt to improve the quality of life of the patient concerned.

8.6 CONCLUSION

This chapter has described the range of therapeutic approaches that can be used with older people. It is suggested that for some it is possible to use standard techniques, although developmental issues will need to be considered as part of an assessment. For some, there will need to be modifications, and Table 8.2 lists some features commonly thought to be helpful. In addition to individual therapeutic approaches, there is an increasing interest in the effectiveness of family therapy. Particular attention has been paid to the analysis of troubling behaviours. Lastly, there are a range of approaches developed especially for use with old people, some concerned with improving the quality of life of dementia sufferers.

It has been one aim of this chapter to illustrate the flexibility with which psychological interventions can be made. Such interventions should be a response to the circumstances of each individual. While it is true that a wide variety of approaches is available, all require careful assessment and thought, while some need extensive training and supervision. Implementing a series of interventions may involve intensive communication between team members and careful delineation of the aims of each. A way of evaluating how far the goals of intervention have been met, and whether or not the intervention has been appropriate, should be part of the treatment. Most interventions and their evaluation should happen within a planned period of time. In this chapter we have also emphasized the responsibility of the therapist for modifying the use of psychological therapy to take account of the special needs of the elderly person. One final word of caution needs to be offered. Psychological approaches will not solve all problems, even when it seems clear that there may be psychological factors. The last case history illustrates just one case where a psychologist was brought in when another form of action would have been more appropriate.

> Case history 8.14:
>
> The patient, Mrs E.R. was referred because she was distressed and spent hours wandering aimlessly in her flat and shouting for help. On assessment, it turned out that she had been discharged from hospital after successful treatment for depression and was awaiting admission into a Residential Home near her daughter. Nothing had happened for some time and Mrs E.R. felt powerless, isolated, depressed and increasingly desperate. In spite of visits from both health and social services, she felt that nothing was being done. The psychologist contacted her social worker, who later discovered that indeed nothing had happened – the referral had somehow been overlooked. Admission was arranged and Mrs E.R. quickly settled.

REFERENCES

1. Segal, H. (1958) Fear of death: notes on the analysis of an old man, in *The Work of Hanna Segal* (1986), Free Association Books and Maresfield Library, London.
2. Colthart, N.E.C. (1991) The analysis of an elderly patient. *International Journal of Psycho-Analysis*, **72**, 209–19.
3. Barraclough, C. and Fleming, I. (1986) *Goal Planning with Elderly People*, Manchester University Press, Manchester.
4. Yost, E. *et al.* (1986) *Group Cognitive Therapy: a Treatment for Depressed Older Adults*, Psychology Practitioner Guidebooks, Pergamon Press, Oxford.
5. Sutton, L. (1991) Reflections on supervision and training in residential homes for elderly people. *British Psychological Society, PSIGE Newsletter*, **39**, 23–6.
6. Hildebrand, H.P. (1982) Psychotherapy with older patients. *British Journal of Medical Psychology*, **55**, 19–28.
7. Knight, R. (1986) *Psychotherapy with the Elderly*, Sage, London.
8. Scrutton, S. (1989) *Counselling Older People*, Age Concern Handbooks, Edward Arnold, London.

9. Carter, B. and McGoldrick, M. (1989) *The Changing Family Life Cycle: a Framework for Family Therapy*, Gardner Press, New York.
10. Holden, U.P. and Woods, R.T. (1988) *Reality Orientation*, 2nd edn, Churchill Livingstone, Edinburgh.
11. Coleman, P. (1986) *Ageing and Reminiscence Processes*, Wiley, London.
12. Morton, I. and Bleathman, C. (1991) The effectiveness of validation therapy in dementia; a pilot study. *International Journal of Geriatric Psychiatry*, **6**, 327–30.
13. Goldstein, A.P. (1980) Relationship-enhancement methods, in *Helping People Change*, (eds F.H. Kanfer and A.P. Goldstein), Pergamon Press, Oxford.
14. Kimmel, D. (1990) *Adulthood and Aging*, Wiley, London.
15. Woods, R.T. and Britton, P.G. (1985) *Clinical Psychology with the Elderly*, Croom Helm, London.
16. Ley, P. (1977) Psychological studies of doctor–patient communication, in *Contributions to Medical Psychology*, (ed. S. Rachman), Pergamon Press, Oxford.
17. King, P. (1974) Notes on the psychoanalysis of older patients. *Journal of Analytic Psychology*, **19**, 22–37.
18. Erikson, E. (1968) *Identity: Youth and Crisis*, Norton, New York.
19. Dershimer, R. (1990) *Counselling the Bereaved*, Psychology Practitioner Guidebooks, Pergamon Press, Oxford.
20. Butler, R.N. (1968) Towards a psychiatry of the life cycle: implications of sociopsychologic studies of the ageing process for the psychotherapeutic situation, *Psychiatric Research Reports*. **23**, 233–48.
21. Herr, J.J. and Weakland, J.H. (1979) *Counselling Elders and their Families: Practical Techniques for Applied Gerontology*, Springer, New York.
22. Brubacker, T. (ed.) (1990) *Family Relationships in Later Life*, 2nd edn, Sage, California.
23. Stokes, G. (1986) *Incontinence and Inappropriate Urinating*, Winslow Press, London.
24. Stokes, G. (1986) *Shouting and Screaming*, Winslow Press, London.
25. Stokes, G. (1986) *Wandering*, Winslow Press, London.
26. Stokes, G. (1986) *Aggression*, Winslow Press, London.
27. Morgan, K. and Gledhill, K. (1991) *Managing Sleep and Insomnia in the Older Person*, Winslow Press, London.
28. Sinason, V. (1992) *Mental Handicap and the Human Condition: New Approaches from the Tavistock*, Free Association Books, London.
29. Butler, R.N. (1963) The life review: an interpretation of reminiscence in the aged. *Psychiatry*, **26**, 65–76.

9

Pharmacological treatment and ECT

Many years ago doctors used to devise their own prescriptions. The symbol used for prescribing, Rx, stands for 'recipe' and many early prescriptions were individual concoctions of various substances. Now, with a wide range of active and standardized drugs, prescribing has a strong scientific basis in the discipline of pharmacology. The emphasis on effective pharmacology has, however, tended to detract from other aspects of treatment, including the relationship between health worker and patient, the reduction of stress for the individual and the family and the provision of a healthy social context. Just as we now have a better understanding of pharmacology, we also have a better understanding of the psychological and social principles of non-pharmaceutical treatment. This has been dealt with in earlier chapters. Here we deal with some of the problems of prescribing medication for old people and some of the principles that can minimize these problems. For convenience we include the treatment of electroplexy in this section.

9.1 SOME OF THE PROBLEMS

A recent British survey of 416 consecutive hospital admissions for old people [1] found that 92 per cent were taking prescribed medication on admission. Forty-eight patients (11.5 per cent) were taking drugs with absolute contra-indications and 113 (27 per cent) patients were taking drugs deemed to be unnecessary. A hundred and three patients (27 per cent) experienced adverse drug reactions and half of these were due to drugs that were either contra-indicated or unnecessary. Twenty-six (6 per cent) admissions were directly attributed to an adverse drug reaction. Diuretics accounted for over half of the adverse effects;

beta-blockers and psychotropics, especially anti-depressants, were the other main offenders. An earlier, larger scale multi-centre study [2] had identified anti-hypertensive drugs, anti-Parkinsonian drugs, psychotropic drugs and diuretics as the most important groups causing adverse reactions which were reckoned to have contributed to about a tenth of admissions. A significant proportion of admissions to psychogeriatric units are precipitated by adverse reactions to medication given for physical as well as psychiatric conditions. Presentations include behaviour disturbance, hypotensive episodes, extrapyramidal symptoms, confusion and excessive sedation [3]. There is an exponential increase in adverse reactions and a linear increase in non-compliance with increasing numbers of drugs prescribed [4]. Nor, of course, are all drugs taken prescribed. An increasing number can be bought 'over the counter' at chemists' shops or drug stores. Elderly women in the UK are, for example, often avid consumers of laxatives. Alcohol is another commonly consumed drug with many interactions with prescribed drugs [5]. While psychotropic drugs can cause physical side-effects, drugs prescribed for physical disease can also cause psychiatric symptoms. Anti-cholinergic drugs, such as benzhexol, still sometimes prescribed for Parkinson's disease but perhaps more often to counteract the side-effects of other drugs, have been shown experimentally to impair memory in old people [6]. L-dopa, bromocriptine and other anti-Parkinsonian drugs can cause psychotic reactions. Many anti-hypertensive drugs can cause psychiatric problems. Digoxin and ACE inhibitors used for cardiovascular disease may cause or maintain depressed mood. Whenever a patient develops psychiatric symtoms, whether depressive, paranoid or confusional, it is essential to review what medication they are receiving.

Prescribing for old people rarely seems to be logical. One general-practice study in the UK showed that 50 per cent of patients over the age of 65 years were receiving repeat prescriptions. On review 62 per cent of these were classed as essential, 28 per cent as equivocal and 10 per cent as definitely unjustified [7]. Another study of over 1000 repeat prescriptions showed that the longer repeat prescribing continued, the less likely it was to be monitored and the more likely the patient was to be elderly [8]. In view of all these problems it is necessary to review the basic facts of drug use in old people.

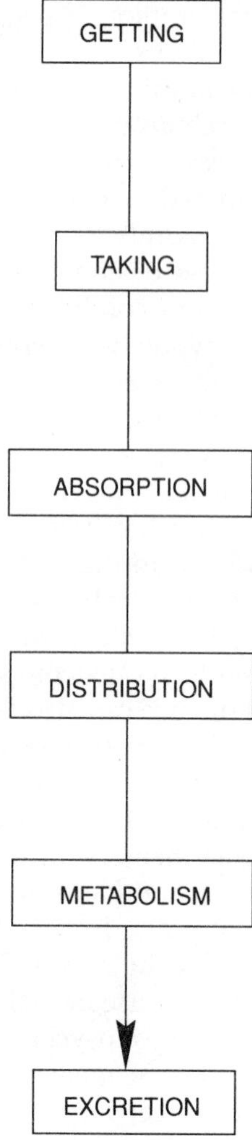

Figure 9.1 Steps in the handling of drugs.

9.2 DRUG HANDLING

Discussions of drug handling usually begin with **absorption**. When dealing with old people, it is important to remember two preliminary steps: getting and taking (see Figure 9.1).

9.2.1 Getting and taking medication

Getting a prescription dispensed is not at all easy for old people. Sadly, doctors on home visits sometimes write a prescription and give no thought as to how the patient will obtain the medication. Sometimes a friend, neighbour or voluntary organization can help, sometimes the doctor needs to pick up the prescription. Often, if the patient can be tided over the first few days with an initial supply given by the doctor, that will give time for someone to get the prescription dispensed. Taking medication is not always that easy. Some old people find childproof safety containers impossible to open [9]. Often the bottles are not labelled in a way that is comprehensible to the patient. Labels with simple, clear instructions are essential and must be in print that is sufficiently large and dense for the patient to read (a condition not often fulfilled by the dot-matrix printers used in many pharmacies). Explaining the medication to the patient, ideally with the tablets in hand for demonstration, is the best way of ensuring that they are taken properly [10]. If drug regimes are complicated, or if the patient is depressed or mildly confused, noting down the purpose of the tablets and when they should be taken on a large card, with samples sellotaped to the card if necessary, can clarify things. Alternatively, for some people, drug drawers which enable a day's medication to be laid out in individually 'timed' drawers can be useful. One chain of pharmaceutical stores in the UK (Boots) has recently started to provide a 'bubble-pack' service with all the medications to be given at a particular time on a particular day of the week laid out in individual labelled press-out bubbles on a card. This device is especially helpful, since it is obvious if a confused patient has been interfering with the medication. There is also a strong case for the education of family members and home-care staff on the sensible management of medication.

Most important, it must never be assumed that, because a drug has been prescribed, it has been taken. Patients sometimes suffer adverse effects when they move into hospital or an old people's home and suddenly start to take drugs which have been prescribed in increasing doses because of apparent ineffectiveness at home which was really due to the patient not taking the drugs. Depot injections, although not ideal for old people for many reasons, are sometimes the only way to be certain that people with schizophrenia receive regular medication.

9.2.2 Absorption

This is the first stage in the conventional metabolism of drugs. It may be slowed by a full stomach or by competition with other drugs. Differences in absorption have not been consistently demonstrated between old and young people.

9.2.3 Distribution

The ratio of lean to fatty tissue decreases with ageing. Many drugs are distributed selectively in lean or fatty tissue. Alcohol is a good example of this and experimental work has shown that after intravenous infusion of a standardized dose of alcohol, old people achieve higher peak serum concentrations, largely because of increased body fat [11]. The lowering of plasma albumin in ill old people can result in the greater availability of drugs which are usually protein-bound.

9.2.4 Sensitivity

The way in which a low blood-potassium level affects the sensitivity of the heart to digoxin has been known for some time but some neuroleptics (e.g. pimozide, droperidol) can also cause arrhythmias in patients with hypokalaemia. The question of the sensitivity of the various brain receptors to psychotropic drugs and how this varies with age, metabolic state and the concurrent administration of other drugs is largely unexplored, although it has been suggested that such increased sensitivity may be the mechanism for the decrease in the intravenous sedative dose of diazepam with increasing age [12].

9.2.5 Metabolism

Most drug metabolism is carried out in the liver. Differences have been found with a slowing of oxidation of chlormethiazole, for example, in some old people. On the other hand, oxidation of some of the benzodiazepines is not impaired. Interactions occur here too. Heavy smoking and alcohol consumption induce enzymes, increasing the speed of metabolism of some drugs. Old people are generally not heavy smokers or drinkers and enzyme induction does not usually occur unless provoked by another prescribed drug. Anti-epileptic drugs can interfere with each other in this way. Liver damage through chronic alcohol abuse produces impaired metabolism. It is important to remember this, for example, when treating withdrawal symptoms in alcoholism with chlormethiazole. Plasma half-life, the time it takes for a drug to decline to half of its peak blood level, is a rough measure of metabolism, though it can be misleading since some drugs are more persistent within the central nervous system than they are in the blood. For many benzodiazepines, plasma half-life is doubled in old age. This can cause accumulation of drugs such as nitrazepam, leading to 'hangover' [13], confusion, unsteadiness and falls. Many drugs (e.g. chlorpromazine) have active metabolic products which make assessment of their handling extremely complicated.

9.2.6 Excretion

Renal function may be impaired in old age. Many drugs or their metabolic products depend on renal excretion for elimination. Some of these can themselves lead to renal impairment. In psychiatry, lithium is the classical example of a drug which is excreted unchanged by the kidneys and where minor upsets in renal function can lead to accumulation and further compromise of renal function with the risk of a potentially fatal vicious circle.

9.3 ADVERSE DRUG REACTIONS

9.3.1 Interactions

The potential for drug interactions is higher in old people because they are such heavy consumers of prescribed drugs. The *British National Formulary* [14] and other formularies have tables of interactions and no attempt will be made to reproduce those here. A few examples will be given to illustrate the problems. Tricyclic anti-depressants and beta-blocking drugs cause postural hypotension. When given together, there can be a profound synergism of these side-effects rendering the patient incapable of standing up without fainting. Case history 4.4 is an example of this. Diuretics ('water tablets'), especially those of the thiazide group, interact with lithium, reducing excretion and carrying a risk of fatal toxicity. If treatment with both drugs is essential, a loop diuretic (e.g. frusemide) is less likely to affect lithium levels but these should still be monitored closely, usually in hospital at first. Conventional mono-amine oxidase inhibitors (MAOIs) interact with certain food and drink, including cheese, yeast extracts, chianti and green banana skins! They also interact in a potentially fatal way with some medications, including the serotonin specific reuptake inhibitor (SSRI) group of anti-depressants as well as with other medications. The SSRIs themselves may cause prolonged fitting with electroplexy (ECT) and may interact with lithium, producing increased serum levels and the risk of toxicity.

Not all interactions are harmful. Patients with resistant depression, unresponsive to anti-depressants alone, sometimes respond to anti-depressants with lithium. In the confused patient who is very disturbed at night, a combination of neuroleptic and hypnotic may sometimes prove a more effective night sedation, with less hangover effect than either drug alone.

9.3.2 Side-effects

Many psychotropic drugs have anti-cholinergic actions. In some neuroleptics like chlorpromazine and thioridazine, the inbuilt anti-cholinergic effects help to neutralize the tendency of the primary action of the drug, dopamine blockade, to cause Parkinsonian symptoms. Anti-cholinergic side-effects generally include dry mouth, blurred vision, constipation and impaired memory. Severe anti-cholinergic side-effects such as glaucoma and urinary retention are relatively rare but important. Dopamine blockade by neuroleptic drugs occasionally causes an acute dystonic reaction. This resembles the occulogyric crisis of post-encephalitic Parkinsonism. The patient's head is suddenly thrown violently back, followed by a phase of relaxation, after which the process may be repeated. This reaction is rare, especially in older people. It sometimes seen after a single dose of a neuroleptic and once seen is never forgotten. It can be aborted by a parenteral dose of procyclidine. More common but slower to develop is the Parkinsonian syndrome with slowing of movements (bradykinesia), loss of associated movements (e.g. arm swinging when walking), tremor (characteristically a 'pill-rolling' tremor, made worse by emotional arousal) and cogwheel rigidity. The best way of treating this is to keep neuroleptic medication to the minimum needed by the patient to live as independently as possible. In elderly schizophrenic patients, a dose of neuroleptic sufficient to suppress symptoms fully will often render the patient completely immobile, and so a suitable compromise between therapeutic and side-effects has to be sought.

Anti-cholinergic drugs should not be used routinely to suppress symptoms caused by neuroleptic drugs since these drugs bring their own side-effects. The longest-term side-effect of neuroleptic treatment is tardive dyskinesia. Restless oro-facial movements with lip-smacking, tongue-rolling and gum-chewing are the commonest symptoms. Larger muscle groups may also be involved. Oro-facial dyskinesia can often be made worse by ill-fitting dentures. Tardive dyskinesia is an unpleasant side-effect that only fades very slowly if the neuroleptic is stopped. There is little effective treatment for it, though it may be temporarily suppressed by increasing neuroleptic dosage. It tends to be worsened by anti-cholinergic drugs. It is best to avoid this complication as far as possible by limiting long-term neuroleptic treatment to those patients for whom it is essential. While neuroleptic drugs are associated with resting and postural tremors, lithium and anti-convulsants tend to produce an action tremor [15]. A rare complication of neuroleptic treatment is **neuroleptic malignant syndrome** with severe muscle rigidity, high temperature and, sometimes, coma and death. It requires hospital treatment.

Anti-depressant side-effects depend on what neurotransmitter systems are predominantly affected. Many of the old tricyclic anti-depressants have strong anti-cholinergic effects (see above) and some have anti-histamine properties which can lead to drowsiness. They may also produce postural hypotension. A **membrane stabilizing** effect is probably responsible for their tendency to cause abnormalities of heart rhythm (sometimes fatal in overdose). The newer serotonin specific reuptake inhibitors (SSRIs) have none of these side-effects but occasionally cause headaches and nausea.

9.3.3 Cost and side-effects

The cost of new drugs makes those responsible for the financial control of the health services exert pressure to use older and cheaper drugs where possible. On the other hand, for the pharmaceutical companies all the profit necessary to support new research and keep the shareholders happy is in new products, before their patent runs out! The clinician is often at the centre of an unhappy tug-of-war between these forces. Most psychotropic drug development in recent years has been a search for selectivity in terms of the neurotransmitter system affected. This tends to produce new drugs with a 'cleaner' pharmacological profile. They are often no more efficacious than earlier drugs, but may target specific symptoms more effectively and usually have fewer side-effects. Some fairly recent psychotropic drug introductions (e.g. zimelidine, nomifensine) were withdrawn because rare but serious side-effects were reported only **after** their introduction to the market.

When evaluating a new drug, the doctor needs to consider the available research evidence for efficacy, side-effects, toxicity in overdose, interactions and cost. Many of the newer anti-depressants, for example, appear to have advantages in side-effects and lack of toxicity which outweigh their extra cost. In addition to the research evidence, most doctors (for better or worse) will be influenced by their personal experience of using a drug. This enables the evaluation of subtle aspects like whether the patients can swallow the preparation (are the tablets too big?) and whether the side-effects that do occur, even if not medically serious, are sufficient to stop the patient taking the medication. It is for this reason that doctors need to develop a personal formulary of drugs. In hospital and general practice, it is now becoming usual to develop a hospital or practice formulary, often with the aim of containing costs.

9.4 A PERSONAL FORMULARY

There are three main groups of drugs in psychiatry: the neuroleptics, the anti-depressants (including lithium) and the 'minor' tranquillizers (most commonly used as sleeping tablets). It is best for doctors to learn a few drugs in each group thoroughly. A personal pharmacopoeia of favourite drugs is given below.

In choosing such a personal formulary, efficacy, side-effects, potential interactions, patient convenience and cost all need to be considered. The list given is far from comprehensive and reflects personal experiences and preferences. For a more comprehensive view, including details of dosage, contra-indications and interactions, the reader is referred to the *British National Formulary* and other appropriate texts.

9.4.1 Neuroleptics

Generally neuroleptics need to be used in lower doses in old people, especially those with organic brain damage. Dosage only needs to be about half that in younger people and dosage intervals can often be longer.

Haloperidol, in higher doses, is an effective neuroleptic for controlling acutely disturbed behaviour. It is a specific and effective treatment for schizophrenia. It has little anti-cholinergic effect and therefore readily induces extrapyramidal ('Parkinsonian') side-effects. It does not usually cause postural hypotension. It is sometimes used in very low doses (0.5–1 mg twice daily) for the treatment of disturbed behaviour in people with dementia, particularly where the disturbance appears to emanate from hallucinations, delusions or other psychotic phenomena. If it is used for longer than a few days, one has to be particularly cautious about extrapyramidal side-effects. There is a very rare but potentially disastrous interaction with lithium [16] which may cause irreversible brain damage. **Trifluoperazine** has a similar profile of action to haloperidol, but is possibly even less sedative. Interactions with lithium are so far not reported.

Thioridazine is a more sedative neuroleptic for the symptomatic control of behavioural disturbance. It has relatively few extrapyramidal effects because of an inbuilt anti-cholinergic effect. It does **not** treat 'confusion'; indeed its sedative and anti-cholinergic effects may worsen confusion. Long-term high-dosage use has occasionally been linked with the serious complication, retinitis pigmentosa, which can cause blindness. **Promazine** is another drug with a similar profile of action, though it is usually regarded as only having a weak anti-psychotic action.

Zuclopenthixol is a sedative neuroleptic, particularly useful in controlling acute disturbance in patients with mania or schizophrenia. It is available in an injectable depot preparation which can be given every two to four weeks to people with schizophrenia if they are not reliable in taking oral medication. There is also an intermediate-acting injectable form (clopixol acuphase) which lasts for two to three days and is a useful way of avoiding repeated intramuscular injections for the acutely disturbed patient who will not take tablets. A disturbed old person generally requires only half the standard dose for younger adults.

Flupenthixol is mainly used as a depot injection for people with schizophrenia. It is not so sedative as zuclopenthixol and may have some mood-elevating properties (it has been marketed in low dose as a safe oral anti-depressant but is not widely used as a 'first line' anti-depressant in hospital practice). The injectable form has been demonstrated to have anti-depressant properties. It remains one of the best depot injections for use in old people because of efficacy combined with a relatively mild extrapyramidal side-effect profile. Depot injections should not normally be used in patients with dementia though they may very occasionally be needed to control disturbed behaviour.

Sulpiride is a partially selective dopamine blocker which sometimes causes fewer extrapyramidal side-effects. It is particularly useful in patients who have intolerable side-effects on other neuroleptics.

Chlorpromazine, the first of the neuroleptics to be discovered, is effective but more sedative, more likely to cause postural hypotension, and more anti-cholinergic than some of the other neuroleptics. Because of its wide spectrum of side-effects it is less often used than the more selective drugs.

Of the above drugs, haloperidol, trifluoperazine, chlorpromazine, promazine and thioridazine are relatively inexpensive.

9.4.2 Anti-depressants

Although we understand something of the biochemical mechanisms by which anti-depressants work, there is much still to be explained, in particular why virtually all anti-depressants have a two- to three-week time lag before their anti-depressant activity begins to manifest itself. Noradrenaline and serotonin depletion are both postulated biochemical mediators of depression. These **neurotransmitters** carry messages across the gap between one nerve-cell and another (the **synaptic cleft**) and are then inactivated by being re-absorbed by the 'sending' cell (**reuptake**). Within the cell, their levels are regulated by **mono-amine oxidases** which break them down into their constituent parts. Many of the older tricyclic anti-depressants (e.g. amitriptyline, imipramine, dothiepin) block serotonin and noradrenaline reuptake, thus increasing their availability in the synaptic cleft, but also have effects on other neurotransmitters (e.g. acetylcholine, histamine) which are responsible for many side-effects. Another less widely used group of drugs, the **mono-amine oxidase inhibitors** (**MAOIs**) cause an accumulation of neurotransmitters by blocking their breakdown. Unfortunately, the original MAOIs also blocked the breakdown of other amines including tyramine, found in many foodstuffs, leading to a potentially fatal raising of blood pressure. Pharmaceutical companies have produced more selective drugs, with fewer unwanted effects.

(a) The serotonin specific reuptake inhibitors (SSRIs)

These relatively new drugs have several different chemical structures and are quite unlike the old tricyclic anti-depressants. They have fewer side-effects and are relatively safe in overdose, though there is a potential of dangerous interaction with MAOIs and a less troublesome interaction with lithium (tendency to increased blood levels, demanding careful monitoring) and ECT (tendency to prolong fit time).

Fluoxetine needs only be taken once a day in a single small capsule and has a long half-life, making it particularly useful where the patient has problems remembering to take the medication. It is not sedative and some patients complain it makes them restless. **Paroxetine and sertraline** both have relatively short half-lives, a useful property in some circumstances (e.g. if it is desired to transfer a patient to a MAOI, the 'washout' period can be shorter), but sometimes require more than a single capsule daily. Paroxetine may be particularly safe in patients with compromised kidney and liver function. The **SSRIs** are relatively expensive.

(b) *Tricyclics*

This class of anti-depressants has many members. Lofepramine is a 'second generation' tricyclic that has relatively weak anti-cholinergic effects and very little anti-histamine or membrane-stabilizing effect. Dry mouth is not usually such a problem as with older tricyclics but constipation can still be a problem. It does not usually cause drowsiness and is remarkably safe in overdose. It blocks reuptake of noradrenaline relatively strongly and thus provides a useful pharmacological contrast to the SSRIs. Dosage is one tablet two or three times a day and the cost is intermediate.

Dothiepin seems to retain the effectiveness of the older tricyclics such as amitriptyline and imipramine with less of the side-effects. It still has relatively strong anti-cholinergic and sedative effects and the majority of the daily dose should be given at night. In order to minimize the side-effects, it is also usual to increase dosage gradually. In overdose, it is, like most other tricyclics, cardiotoxic and should be used with caution in people with known arrhythmias or high risk of overdose. It will probably be gradually displaced by newer, safer drugs. It is relatively cheap, though not as inexpensive as amitriptyline and imipramine which are not widely used in psychogeriatric practice.

(c) *Mono-amine oxidase inhibitors (MAOIs)*

Phenelzine can be effective in patients with mixed anxiety and depressive symptoms. It calls for dietary and drug restrictions and the patient should be told about these and should always carry a warning card. Its effect in appropriate subjects is dramatic and it has been shown to be effective in long-term prophylaxis. Perhaps for this reason, once started, the treatment is very hard to withdraw without relapse. A new class of MAOIs, free of the 'cheese reaction' (and other interactions) is in development and the first of these, **moclobamide**, is already available.

(d) *Lithium carbonate*

This is especially effective in prophylaxis of manic-depressive and recurrent depressive illness. The commonest side-effects are an increased fluid intake and urine output, a mild tremor and, long-term, some inhibition of thyroid function, sometimes requiring supplementary treatment with thyroxine. This drug has a low therapeutic margin and serum levels must be carefully monitored, initially weekly and eventually monthly or three-monthly. Nowadays levels are usually kept around 0.4–0.5 in old people. Good renal function is a prerequisite to treatment [17] and thyroid function should be checked every few months. Sometimes patients who do not respond to one of the other anti-depressants alone will respond to a combination of the antidepressant with lithium. Patients on lithium should be warned about the risks of toxicity and told to stop the treatment immediately if they develop nausea, diarrhoea, vomiting or if they are otherwise unwell. They should report this immediately to their doctor who can advise them when to re-start the medication. Printed cards with a warning about side-effects and toxicity are available, and can be very useful (Figure 9.2).

9.4.3 'Minor' tranquillizers and hypnotics

(a) Benzodiazepines

Generally drugs of this group are best avoided in old people. If relaxation is needed, it should be provided by appropriate social or psychological therapy (see Chapter 8), rather than by drugs.

Diazepam. One of the earliest benzodiazepines and one of the cheapest, this drug has an extended half-life in old people and dosage should be kept low and limited to short courses. It is usually given by mouth for anxiety but has an occasional use in very severely demented patients with muscle spasm because of its muscle-relaxant effects.

Lormetazepam. At present, this seems to be one of the best hypnotics for old people. It is a small tablet, easy to take and has an intermediate half-life with little hangover or cumulative effect, providing the dosage is kept low. **Nitrazepam** is best avoided in old people because of the risks of accumulation and **temazepam** is harder to take than lormetazepam, sometimes too short-acting with wakening in the middle of the night and, occasionally, it seems to produce the need for increasing dose and a risk of dependency. All the benzodiazepines carry this

Lithium Treatment Card

ALWAYS CARRY THIS CARD WITH YOU

If you become ill from whatever cause and require a doctor please show him this card.

Name ....

Address ....

....

....

Clinic...

Telephone ....

Doctor...

Lithium is a treatment used to prevent excessive mood swings, and to be effective must be taken regularly. Remember that you should continue taking your tablets as your doctor directs even though you feel perfectly well.

The following notes are for your guidance:—

1. Take the tablets regularly at the same time each day as directed by your doctor. The dose has been selected individually to suit you.
2. The dose may need adjusting in the first few weeks of treatment and this is judged by your blood test results. On the day of your blood test do not take your tablets until after the test.
3. Like most medicines, lithium carbonate may have some 'side effects'. Usually these will last only for a short time.
4. Tell your doctor at once if you have any of the following:—
   diarrhoea or vomiting
   giddiness or loss of balance
   abnormal drowsiness
   severe trembling of hands or feet
   excessive thirst
   increased urination.
5. The doctor will want to see you from time to time to check your progress and to make sure that your dose remains correct.

The reverse of this card carries a table with spaces for appointments, dose of lithium and serum levels.

Figure 9.2 Lithium card.

risk to a greater or lesser degree and in patients who have been receiving them for some time, they should be discontinued gradually, to avoid withdrawal symptoms. Patients who have been on long-term benzodiazepines sometimes develop memory problems and may become acutely anxious or depressed on withdrawal, which may have to be conducted on an inpatient basis.

(b) Others

Chlormethiazole is an effective night sedative and can be used to reduce daytime agitation in confused patients, especially those who react adversely to a neuroleptic such as thioridazine. It is available either in capsule or liquid form. The patient may find the liquid preparation rather unpleasant-tasting though this can sometimes be disguised with orange juice. Chlormethiazole has a use in a decreasing dose regime to prevent the development of **delerium tremens** in alcohol withdrawal. Long-term use should be avoided because of the risk of dependence.

9.4.4 Electroplexy (Electro-convulsive therapy, ECT)

This is the treatment of choice for severely depressed patients, especially if life is threatened by dehydration or suicide. It is also particularly indicated where there is marked depressive psychomotor slowing (retardation) or where delusions are part of the clinical picture. Prognosis of severe depression may be improved by the use of ECT [18]. Unilateral non-dominant treatment twice weekly used to be recommended as less likely to cause memory problems, though there is some evidence that bilateral treatment may be more rapidly effective. Newer ECT machines minimize side-effects and thrice-weekly bilateral treatment is now being increasingly used in younger adults, though there is not yet enough experience to recommend this in older patients. Memory problems are usually transient and less severe than those caused by the depression itself. The patient is anaesthetized and given a muscle relaxant to modify the fit. It is essential that ECT is followed by anti-depressant or lithium therapy to minimize the risk of relapse. Because of 'bad press', ECT may be given less often than it should be at present.

The above is a brief list of the treatments most commonly

used by one of the authors. It is not intended to be exhaustive and many details such as dosage, interactions and some side-effects, have been omitted. The list emphasizes that a relatively small group of drugs can cover most psychiatric situations and raises the issue of whether newer, more expensive drugs with fewer (known) side-effects are to be preferred over older, cheaper and more unpleasant or dangerous drugs. The latest is not necessarily the best but where it presents a significant increase in safety, it should always be considered.

9.5 THE PRINCIPLE OF MINIMAL MEDICATION

Stated briefly, this principle is that old people should always be given the minimal amount of medication needed to treat their illness or alleviate their suffering. Alternatives to drug treatment should always be sought. A good example of this is the patient who complains of poor sleep (insomnia). This may be symptomatic (e.g. early morning wakening in depressive illness or paroxysmal nocturnal dyspnoea in heart failure) and, if so, it should be treated appropriately. On the other hand, the patient may have unrealistic expectations. The total amount of sleep needed seems to decrease with increasing age [19] especially if the patient takes little exercise and 'catnaps' through the day, and the patient may not realize this. Non-pharmaceutical measures should precede any use of medication. More exercise, more interesting activity during the day, excluding 'catnaps' and the traditional warm milky drink at night, can all be tried. On the other hand, if the patient is drinking too much in the afternoon and evening, especially if the drinks contain stimulants like caffeine or diuretics like caffeine and alcohol, then sleep may be interfered with by over-stimulation or the need to rise repeatedly to go to the toilet. Drinking may have to be restricted. The management of insomnia in the confused patient has been discussed briefly in Chapter 5 and illustrated in Figure 5.4., and the general psychological management of insomnia has been considered in Chapter 2. Another common symptom that responds better to rational analysis than symptomatic prescribing is incontinence, as described in Chapter 8 and illustrated here in Case history 9.1.

Case history 9.1:

Mrs B.Y. was a 93-year-old widow who lived alone in an old back-to-back terraced house. Her mobility had become restricted and she had started to sleep in her downstairs room which was a combined living room and kitchen. Her toilet was down two flights of outside stairs in the cellar. She became incontinent because of difficulty in reaching the toilet and a commode was provided but she refused to use it, saying (quite reasonably) that it did not flush and was in her kitchen. She was referred to the psychogeriatric service because of confusion and incontinence. She had mild intellectual impairment but gave logical reasons for not using the commode. When admitted to day hospital, she behaved quite appropriately, going to the toilet and using it readily. Because of a multitude of problems, her adjustment at home was poor and she was admitted to residential care where she continued to be continent. Her incontinence was almost entirely situational in cause.

This case illustrates how important environmental factors can be in the causation and management of incontinence. Equally a local cause such as urinary infection, retention (possibly caused by drugs) or severe constipation may be responsible for incontinence. Only when these and other causes have been excluded should a **symptomatic** pharmacological approach be considered.

The **symptomatic** use of drugs, for example the use of neuroleptics to control disturbed behaviour, or a hypnotic at night, should be distinguished from their **specific** use (e.g. neuroleptics for schizophrenia or anti-depressants for depressive episodes). When drugs are being used symptomatically, it is especially important to seek alternatives and limit the length of treatment. When drugs must be used, then the principle of minimal medication means that the **smallest possible number** of drugs should be used at any one time in the **smallest effective dose** for the **shortest time necessary for effective treatment**. This principle is summarized in Table 9.1.

Table 9.1 The principle of minimal medication

1. Seek alternatives
2. Distinguish specific from symptomatic treatment
3. Give the smallest number of drugs
4. In the lowest effective dose
5. For the shortest time needed

Some drugs, such as anti-depressants, may need to be given for at least 6–12 months or indefinitely if there are recurrent attacks. Similarly schizophrenic patients may need a lifetime prescription of neuroleptics. In these cases it is especially important to choose drugs with the minimum of unwanted effects and to monitor their usage carefully, as there may be a need to decrease the dose with increasing age.

This chapter stresses the risks of careless prescribing. Pills are only one of the doctor's therapeutic options. In conjunction with other disciplines, psychological and social help can and should be offered when appropriate. Using a neuroleptic to sedate a confused elderly patient at home or on a long-stay ward because of under-staffing or service inadequacies is little different in principle to the abuse of psychotropic drugs to control political dissenters in some countries. Both involve the use of chemical agents to hide or compensate for social deficiencies. Doctors should not fall into this trap. However, we must not over-react against drugs. We must remember that, properly used, psychotropic drugs can cure illness, alleviate suffering and even save life. A further discussion of drug treatment for the elderly mentally ill can be found in the *Handbook of Geriatric Psychopharmacology* [20].

REFERENCES

1. Lindley, C.M., Tully, M.P., Paramsothy, V. and Tallis, R.C. (1992) Inappropriate medication is a major cause of adverse drug reactions in elderly patients. *Age and Ageing*, **21**, 294–300.
2. Williamson, J. and Chopin, J.M. (1980) Adverse reactions to prescribed drugs in the elderly: a multi-centre investigation. *Age and Ageing*, **9**, 73–80.
3. Briant, R.H. (1977) Drug treatment in the elderly: problems and prescribing rules. *Drugs*, **13**, 225–9.

4. Castleden, C.M. (1978) Prescribing for the elderly. *Prescriber's Journal*, **18**, 90–4.
5. Anonymous leader (1980) Drugs and alcohol. *British Medical Journal*, **i**, 507–8.
6. Potamianos, G. and Kellett, J.M. (1982) Anticholinergic drugs and memory: the effects of benzhexol on memory in a group of geriatric patients. *British Journal of Psychiatry*, **140**, 470–2.
7. Tulloch, A.J. (1981) Repeat prescribing for elderly patients. *British Medical Journal*, **282**, 1672–5.
8. Dennis, P.J. (1979) Monitoring of psychotropic drug prescribing in general practice. *British Medical Journal*, **ii**, 115–16.
9. Sherman, F.T., Warach, J.D. and Libow, L.S. (1979) Child-resistant containers for the elderly. *Journal of the American Medical Association*, **241**, 1001–2.
10. McDonald, E., McDonald, J.B. and Phoeni, M. (1977) Improving drug compliance after discharge. *British Medical Journal*, **ii**, 618–21.
11. Vestal, R.E., McGuire, E.A., Tobin, J.D. *et al.* (1977) Ageing and ethanol metabolism in man. *Clinical Pharmacology and Therapeutics*, **3**, 343–54.
12. Cook, P.J., Flanagan, R. and James, I.M. (1984) Diazepam tolerance: effect of age, regular sedation and alcohol. *British Medical Journal*, **289**, 351–3.
13. Cook, P.J., Huggett, A., Graham-Pole, R. *et al.* (1983) Hypnotic accumulation and hangover in elderly inpatients: a controlled doubleblind study of temazepam and nitrazepam. *British Medical Journal*, **286**, 100–2.
14. *The British National Formulary* (1992) The British Medical Association and the Royal Pharmaceutical Society of Great Britain.
15. Lane, R.J. (1984) Drugs and tremor. *Adverse Drug Reactions Bulletin*, **106**, 392–5.
16. Thomas, C.J. (1979) Brain damage with lithium and haloperidol (letter). *British Journal of Psychiatry*, **134**, 552.
17. Hansen, H.E. (1981) Renal toxicity of lithium. *Drugs*, **22**, 461–76.
18. Baldwin, R. (1988) Late-life depression: undertreated (leader). *British Medical Journal*, **296**, 519.
19. Quan, S.F., Bamford, C.R. and Beutler, L.E. (1985) Insomnia. *Geriatric Medicine*, **15**, 11–15.
20. Jenike, M.A. (1985) *A Handbook of Geriatric Psychopharmacology*, PSG Publishing Company, Littleton, Massachusetts.

10

The organization of services and the law in relation to treatment

Although the United Kingdom took a lead in the development of specialist psychiatric services for old people, other countries have developed their own models depending on the way in which health and social care is organized locally. The authors' experience is chiefly in the United Kingdom and it is mostly to experience in that country that we will refer, though many of the principles involved can be generalized to other settings.

10.1 PLANNING A PSYCHIATRIC SERVICE FOR OLD PEOPLE

The **clinical** functions of a comprehensive psychiatric service for old people can be broken down into four compartments:

assessment and communication;
community treatment and support;
acute inpatient treatment;
long-stay residential/nursing care (see Figure 10.1).

In addition, a comprehensive service will also have a training and educational role and should be involved in research and development and audit, if only at a local level, to ensure that the best possible quality is achieved for the resources invested.

10.1.1 A balanced service

Clinical assessment is the key to an effective service. It involves a comprehensive evaluation of the person's physical, psychiatric and social needs, and should be thorough at the point of entry to the system and whenever needs change or a move from one

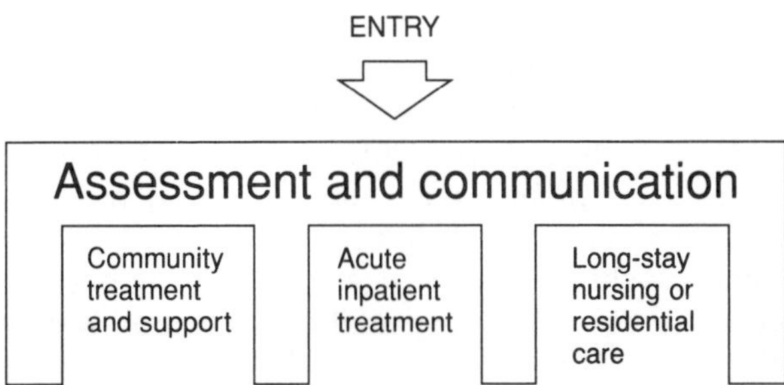

Figure 10.1 Functions of a psychiatric service for old people.

compartment of care to another is envisaged. Assessment must be coupled to good **communication** both internally and with others concerned in providing care for the patient. Systems which have inadequate assessment may, for example, provide expensive long-term care for people who, had they been adequately assessed, might only have needed a short period of medical treatment. Systems with inadequate acute or long-stay institutional care throw undue strain on staff involved in community treatment and support. As these staff are, or often should be, involved in assessment, this strain may further compromise the assessment function, perhaps leading to a breakdown in the whole system, to the detriment of all old people who need the service. Weakness in community-support facilities can overload acute inpatient facilities, and lack of long-stay care can block exit from acute inpatient facilities. In planning, therefore, the whole assessment, treatment and support network must be seen as an interactive system.

10.1.2 Target population

Until 1992, in the UK it was reckoned that one consultant and the associated team of workers could cope effectively with an area containing about 22 000 old people [1]. This assumed a comprehensive service which dealt with all mental illness in old people (possibly excepting those who had grown old in hospital) and not the much rarer pattern of a dementia-only service. With the increasing proportion of very old people and the higher expectations placed on services, the Royal College of Psychiatrists has recently recommended that the number served by one consultant should be reduced to 10 000 old people [2]. In addition the College has suggested that, in teaching health districts, where staff have extra educational responsibilities, catchment areas should be commensurately smaller. In Australia, with its lower proportion of older people, one general psychiatrist has suggested that only one specialist psychiatrist for the elderly per million population is needed, a suggestion hotly contested by Australian psychogeriatricians [3]! The total population served must also be known in order to decide what personnel and facilities (for example, day-hospital places and inpatient beds) are needed. Whatever the size of population served, it is usually agreed that a restricted geographical area should be chosen, because this enables the team to build up relationships with other local workers and to become familiar with the network of facilities available locally. In the UK, General Practitioners, district nurses, social workers, home helps and other social and voluntary workers and the day-care, lunch-club, carer support and other services they provide, are important local relationships. The recent reorganization of the National Health Service has put a premium on competition and market forces and it remains to be seen how far this will change current patterns of service.

10.1.3 Integrated care

Care of the elderly is an area where the traditional distinction between care in the community and hospital-based care is inadequate. Although General Practitioners and area social services workers act as the first line of contact for services in the community, hospital-based teams pride themselves on providing many diagnostic and treatment services to the patient at home. Whereas in some areas of general psychiatry, Community Mental Health teams have grown up almost independent of the hospital services, in old-age psychiatry a more 'integrated' model is often found, with the same core team of people involved in assessing and managing the patient in the community as are responsible for inpatient or day-patient care. This model has avoided some of the problems of Community Mental Health teams, especially the tendency for the community team to provide fewer services for those with serious mental illness and more for those with relatively minor problems. The old idea that care in the community was entirely the prerogative of the general practitioner has been re-evaluated. The hospital-based psychiatrist is much more than just a 'gate-keeper' for admission to inpatient or day-hospital facilities. The specialist team needs to work in co-operation with General Practitioners and area social services to set up adequate networks of care for old people with psychiatric illness in the community.

10.1.4 The team

The typical specialist team consists of a consultant and one or more doctors in training as well as community nurses, and contributions from one or more social workers, occupational therapist(s), physiotherapist(s), ward- and day-hospital nurses and psychologist(s). Inequalities in health care from one place to another are nowhere more evident than in the field of specialist psychiatric services for old people [4].

10.1.5 Facilities

These include day-hospital places, acute beds and long-stay beds. The best team in the world can do little if not backed by appropriate facilities. In the UK, the Royal College of Psychiatrists [1, 2] and the Department of Health and Social Security [5] have both suggested guidelines for psychiatric services for the elderly and the Health Advisory Service [6] and a joint report of the Royal Colleges of Psychiatrists and Physicians [7] have reiterated some of these. Guidelines are summarized in Table 10.1.

Table 10.1 Guidelines for special provision for mentally ill old people (per 1000 population greater than 65 years)

Acute assessment and treatment beds	1.5
Day-hospital places (dementia and share of non-dementia places)	2.65–3.65
Long-stay beds for demented old people	2.5–3

(Sources: Royal College of Psychiatrists; Department of Health and Social Security [1, 5])

(a) Day-hospital facilities

These form part of the community-treatment resource. Their importance and how they are used varies from locality to locality. They may serve several different functions. Some places are used for assessment, some to support severely demented people whose relatives want to keep them at home but who need a regular 'break'. Others are used to support those who are in need of 24-hour care while they wait for a place to become available in hospital or in a residential or nursing home. They are not solely used for people with dementia. Many of the patients are suffering from recurrent depressive disorder and some from paranoid disorders, alcohol abuse or other problems. For them, day-hospital treatment may avoid the need for inpatient care or may enable patients to be discharged home sooner and kept in relatively good health despite social isolation and other unfavourable circumstances.

The effective functioning of day hospitals depends upon the provision of other facilities such as social services and voluntary Day Centres, to which those patients who need it can be discharged for 'social' maintenance. Transport is also a vital factor in day hospitals as most patients cannot make their own way to the hospital and transport services need to be arranged so that it is possible for them to wait a while for those who are not ready when the vehicle calls. Relatives, home helps, district nurses, community nurses and others may need to be enlisted to make sure that the old person does attend the day-hospital facility. In geographically compact areas, day hospitals whose primary function is assessment, treatment and rehabilitation are probably best located, together with acute beds, in the district general hospital. Day hospitals providing continuing support for behaviourally disturbed people with dementia could well be distributed with long-stay beds throughout the community served, though this model may be under threat in the UK at present with the move away from planned provision to a 'quasi-market' approach, of opportunistic provision in the private sector. In some areas of relatively scattered populations, the 'mobile' day hospital has been developed. Staff and equipment travel from the base hospital to a different location each day and run a day hospital in a local church hall, community centre or other suitable facility. This is a useful way of spreading thin resources across a wide geographical area. Another model, yet to be tried on any scale, is the provision of health-service staff to provide extended short-term home care as an alternative to admission or day-hospital assessment, perhaps in association with local authority Day Centres.

Few services approach the guidelines for day places given by the Department of Health, and many acknowledge that these guidelines were over-generous. Provided that social services and voluntary facilities for day care and other community care are adequate, a smaller number of day-hospital places can concentrate on the assessment and treatment of people with functional illness, preventing or curtailing inpatient care and on the assessment of particular diagnostic or behavioural problems in people with dementia. In our own area, long-term day care is mostly provided by the social services, with the Alzheimer's Disease Society taking an increasing role, though the hospital service still takes a few people that other facilities cannot manage.

(b) Acute inpatient facilities

These can be located on one ward for all different types of mental illness, although services increasingly provide separate wards for the assessment of those who are markedly confused, and for the treatment of other disorders. The location of acute assessment beds is as important as their number. Because of frequent concurrent physical illness and the need for ready access to investigative facilities and close co-operation with geriatric medicine, these beds are best located on a general hospital site where they can be used more efficiently.

(c) Respite care

Respite can help relatives to continue coping in the community. Patients come in for a pre-arranged stay at regular intervals or to cover special needs like annual holidays. Some respite care for people with dementia was traditionally offered in social services homes and, for the severely disabled, some care was offered in psychogeriatric or geriatric hospital beds, depending on whether the disability was predominantly behavioural or physical. The reduction of beds across the public sector has led to a loss of these services in some areas and in many cases, the private sector has not found it commercially feasible to fill this gap. Hopefully new purchasing arrangements with the private sector will make an enhanced provision of respite care available. Respite care does not help all patients with dementia. Some exhibit increased confusion and hostility during and after a respite admission.

(d) Continuing care

Long-stay beds for elderly demented people are still often located in the old mental hospitals. These are now far fewer than were available when the first edition of this book was published, since the government has promoted the expansion of private long-stay provision, effectively at the expense of NHS care. Continuing care facilities are essential for people with severe dementia who need 24-hour care which cannot always be provided in their own homes. From the end of the Second World War until the mid-1980s a policy evolved in the UK which broadly divided those with dementia into three groups. Those who were immobile went to NHS geriatric facilities, those who were mobile and without major behavioural problems were looked after at home or in social services 'part III' accommodation, and those who had major behavioural problems were cared for in psychiatric facilities. The private sector was not interested in these difficult patients. Then the DHSS changed its benefit rules which encouraged a rapid expansion of private sector provision at public expense. The Audit Commission reviewed the situation. The result, incorporated in the Community Care Act, was a measure to 'cap' this spending by transferring money from the benefit system (in April 1993) into an unspecified but **limited** fund administered through local government authorities which are expected to **assess** people before placement in residential or **nursing** homes.

Two basic premises underlie this reform. The first is that making the same authority responsible for residential, nursing and community care will remove perverse financial incentives to move people into residential- and nursing-home care who could be looked after in the community. The second is that people going into care at the public expense should be properly assessed. Even now, most people who go into care need it. Virtually all those people placed from geriatric or psychogeriatric services are already carefully assessed. Close co-operation between health and social services, especially in social services accepting assessments already made by health-service multidisciplinary teams, will be essential to avoid 'demarcation' disputes over people needing nursing care. Agreement over which of those people who need nursing care should receive it in the health-service sector will probably be based more upon the need for active medical or psychiatric attention and difficult behaviour rather than on overall levels of disability. We collected data on dementia and disability levels in samples of residential, nursing home and psychogeriatric care [8] in Leeds. We excluded geriatric care because we could not identify specific 'long-stay' care settings. We estimated the number of people with dementia and in each disability category in each setting. We found dementia in 97 per cent of the residents in hospital and local authority specialist homes for the 'elderly mentally infirm' (EMI), 93 per cent of the residents in registered mental nursing homes, 80 per cent of the people in local authority residential homes and 59 per cent of residents in private residential care. Dementia was associated with higher overall levels of disability.

Residential and general nursing homes contained a small proportion (12 per cent) of people with low disability, though less than 5 per cent were likely to be capable of 'independent' living. Local authority EMI homes, registered mental nursing homes and psychogeriatric beds only contained people in the three highest dependency grades and predominantly in the highest of these.

We estimated there were 3400 people in the two highest dependency grades in Leeds, a city of around 800 000 total population, who could be classed as clearly needing nursing care. Only the minority of these currently receive care from the health service and it will be important to develop explicit criteria to identify those who should receive 'free' health provision and those who should be cared for in means-tested nursing home provision purchased by local government. If funding is inadequate the total 'pool' of care will not match the needs of the population.

The intention of the government to separate 'purchaser' and

'provider' of health care and to increase provision in the private sector has been coupled with initiatives to establish a code of care [9] and monitoring by local health and social services authorities which should help ensure quality; but the quality of **care** as opposed to the quality of the **environment** is costly to measure in an objective way. However, methods do exist, including a promising technique called 'dementia care mapping' [10] which is based on observation of interactions and activity by trained raters. Only with methods like this will we be able to get a true assessment of quality.

The health-care system in the USA is quite different. There is less emphasis on the 'primary care' function of general practitioners and private facilities provide much of the acute and continuing psychiatric care for old people. These are supported by private health-insurance schemes and, for the poor, by social security legislation. The net result is that the USA has some of the finest acute and long-stay facilities in the world, but their availability is even more constrained by geographical and financial considerations than in the UK. For a fuller discussion of the system of health care for the elderly in the USA and its funding the reader is referred to the *Core of Geriatric Medicine* [11].

10.2 SOCIAL SERVICES PROVISION

The vast majority of mentally ill old people live at home. If they are lonely or dependent for basic needs on others, then social services provision is often appropriate. Other forms of help have been recently added to the traditional pattern of home-care workers, meals-on-wheels and laundry services. The neighbourhood warden, who is paid by social services to provide a daily human contact for old people living alone, and family-placement schemes where families are paid to take in old people, often to give their caring relatives a break, are two examples. Trained social workers are also beginning to take a greater interest in the personal needs of old people and their carers, though legislation ensures that most skilled social worker time is spent on child care. Community services are now more often available in the evenings and at weekends, though there are still often yawning gaps during public holidays. Special out-of-hours services such as night sitting are only patchily available. The majority of provision is still by social services, although 'Crossroads' and other care schemes provided by voluntary bodies often pioneer new services on a small scale.

10.3 BOUNDARIES

In the UK, when old people need medical treatment, it is clearly the province of the General Practitioner or the hospital authorities. When they need community services such as home care or meals-on-wheels, it is largely the responsibility of local government-controlled social services although district nurses and community psychiatric nurses often contribute.

Providers of health services and social services in the UK are now required by government to institute a **care-planning procedure** [12]. This is intended to be a monitorable mechanism by which joint care plans are drawn up for people receiving help from more than one agency. Workers from all agencies, the patient and his or her relatives or caregivers, are involved in the process of producing a care plan which meets the patient's perceived need, which is reviewed regularly and which has 'shared ownership'. Unfortunately, given the low priority accorded to skilled work with old people in some social services departments and the limited resources available in psychogeriatric services, the time is rarely available to carry out these procedures in a way that is satisfactory. The **case-management approach** is about to be introduced in social services. Hopefully this will be more flexible and efficient than the previous piecemeal approach to provision that prevailed in some areas – but only if sufficient resources are made available to provide the services as well as plan and manage them!

For those who need residential/nursing-home care, the best solution might well be a combined care facility where staff were available to cope with all levels of disability. People admitted to such a facility would be able to stay there for the rest of their lives and still get increased levels of nursing care should they need it. This is the pattern of care provided, for example, in some parts of Australia, where residential care facilities often have their own 'nursing home' on the same site. There has been no attempt to provide this kind of care systematically in the United Kingdom and divided responsibilities with local authority housing departments or voluntary bodies responsible for sheltered housing, social services departments responsible for purchasing (means-tested) residential care and nursing-home care and the National Health Service responsible for providing free nursing care, militate against it!

10.4 VOLUNTARY PROVISION

Some of the finest initiatives in the care of elderly people with psychiatric disorders are in the 'voluntary' sector. Housing associations provide sheltered housing which will often help alleviate the loneliness of the depressed old person or enable a husband/wife to continue looking after a demented spouse. Groups of relatives of elderly mentally ill people meet for mutual support and have, in some areas, arranged sophisticated day-care facilities. Volunteers in 'good neighbour schemes', 'Crossroads' or 'care groups' do the shopping or sit with elderly patients at home while relatives take a break. In the USA and Australia voluntary and charitable bodies, often with church associations, have played a much more prominent role in developing nursing home, residential home and other facilities for long-term care and support of old people than in the UK, though there have been some notable initiatives from the Church of Scotland. Other schemes, such as the family-placement scheme in Leeds, are organized by social services with payment to a family to take in old people usually for a few weeks at a time while the regular carers take a holiday.

10.5 MULTI-DISCIPLINARY WORKING

The involvement of different organizations and different disciplines in work for old people with mental illness provides an opportunity for creative co-operation if the workers and their respective organizations can get along together. If they cannot manage to do this, whole groups of elderly people can be left 'out in the cold' as health and social services dispute who is responsible. Most psychiatric services for old people are based on a team of people from different disciplines who, as well as providing services directly, also liaise with many other people outside the 'core' team. Patterns of working together vary widely from team to team and from time to time within a team.

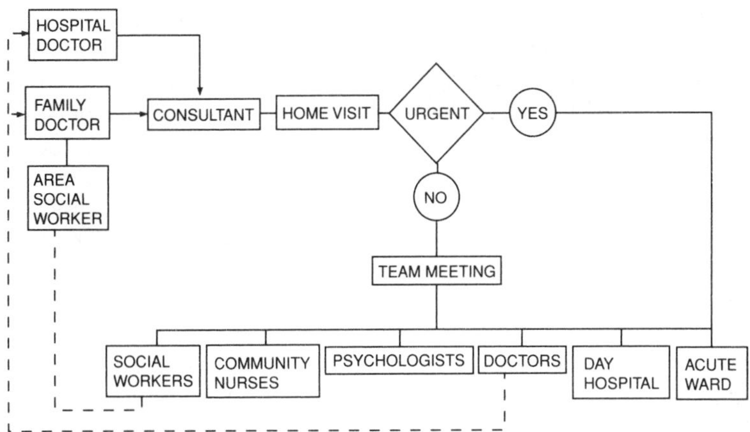

Figure 10.2 Flow chart illustrating the working of a particular specialist psychiatric team.

The following description illustrates how the team with which the authors are familiar functions at present. The method of dealing with new referrals is illustrated in the flow chart in Figure 10.2.

New referrals come, usually from the patient's family doctor (General Practitioner) to the consultant or his secretary. About a quarter of referrals are from other hospital doctors and some 'community' referrals are really initiated by social service personnel with the approval of the appropriate General Practitioner. Sometimes team members take direct referrals from or give informal advice to social workers or care staff about a particular problem. Medical responsibility for these people remains with the GP unless a referral has been made to the psychiatrist with the GP's approval, when medical responsibility for patients who remain in the community is shared between consultant and GP. Once a patient has been referred medically, he or she is seen at home by a senior psychiatrist (consultant or senior registrar) and an initial assessment is made. This normally happens within a few hours for urgent referrals and usually within a few days for less urgent cases. If the assessment indicates that urgent action is needed, the assessing doctor initiates this immediately. All cases are discussed at the weekly team meeting where the different disciplines have a chance to comment and make suggestions about management. Once a member of the team accepts responsibility for a particular patient in the community, that person becomes, regardless of discipline, the 'contact person' for those outside the team and is, as far as possible, the focus for any further management decisions. The team meeting also provides an opportunity for members of the team to present ongoing cases with whom they are having particular difficulties for group discussion and possibly to enlist the help of other disciplines in coping with the problem.

Some patients are assessed to be in need of urgent physical rather than psychiatric attention. They are referred back to the family doctor or to the appropriate medical specialist (usually the physician in geriatric medicine). Many patients who are referred will be already known to local social-work staff who may be invited to participate in meetings where their clients are to be reviewed and are generally kept in touch with how the team is managing their clients. Referrals to non-medical team members are assessed by the appropriate discipline. If the management plan produced requires help from other members of the team, especially medical staff, this is negotiated with GPs, who understand our team's multi-disciplinary style of working. This flexible pattern of working makes it extremely difficult to put a true price on our services in the new 'internal market' that exists with fund-holding GPs and purchasing health authorities.

For successful multi-disciplinary working, there has to be a sense of trust and mutual respect between team members. Because of the markedly different training between different disciplines, this can be hard to achieve. There are overlapping areas of expertise and it is only by discussing case management frankly together that the most appropriate skills can be applied to a particular patient's problems. One model for understanding the overlap between different disciplines is presented in Figure 10.3.

Each discipline has its area of expertise. For example, area A in the doctor's portion of the figure represents such things as medical diagnosis and the prescribing of drugs where only the doctor has the appropriate training and skills. A similar area for the nurse might be the planned provision of 24-hour care to support patients and at the same time help them to develop

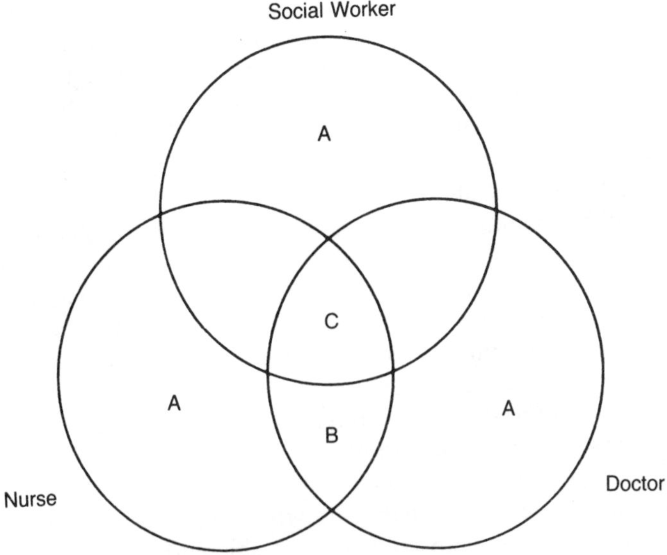

Figure 10.3 Overlaps of skill in the multi-disciplinary team.

their own self-care skills; or for the home-care manager or social worker, the detailed planning and provision of support services in the community. Other areas of skill and responsibility overlap (B). A simple example of this is the giving of injections where both doctors and nurses have appropriate training. Yet other areas (C) may be shared by all members of the team. All disciplines, for example, might have training in bereavement counselling. The diagram is oversimplified but still gives some idea of the complexity of multi-disciplinary working. The psychologist on the team may have special skills in neuropsychological and behavioural assessment but also share some skills in counselling or psychotherapy with other disciplines. The same mixture of unique and shared skills is also found in occupational therapy, physiotherapy and other disciplines. The exact areas of overlap in any team will depend not only on boundaries between disciplines, but also on individual training and talent. What is important is that the areas of unique skill or responsibility and of overlap are recognized and that team members are prepared to accept each other's skills, regardless of different training backgrounds. Members of the team must also guard against the tendency to concentrate on the more 'interesting' aspects of work while the more mundane tasks are left undone, and be secure enough in their own work to listen to constructive criticism from other disciplines. If such an ethos can be achieved, mistakes in planning care will be minimized, as all members of the team will be enabled to contribute responsibly.

Another potential source of conflict in multi-disciplinary working is the different hierarchical structure of different disciplines illustrated in Figure 10.4. This figure, again, is an over-simplification, as only three disciplines are included. Medicine is the only discipline where authority rests more or less absolutely with the most senior clinical member of the team. Other disciplines have to rely, to varying degrees, on the decisions of more senior members of their disciplines who are not involved in the day-to-day clinical working of the team. If they have good higher managers who are prepared to delegate authority and the team members are able and willing to accept this, then everything can work well. If this delegation cannot be achieved, for whatever reason, true multi-disciplinary working is hard to achieve.

Leadership is a vital function within the team. The overall leader is usually the consultant psychiatrist but problems arise

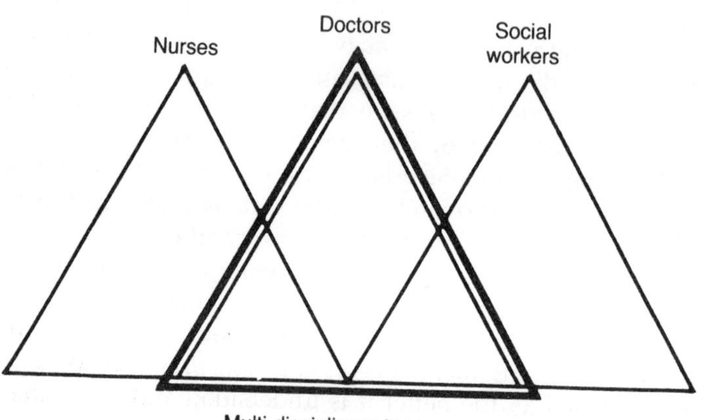

Figure 10.4 Hierarchical professional structures and the multi-disciplinary team.

when he or she does not possess the necessary skills or when another member of the team is *de facto* the leader while the consultant remains **nominally** in charge. The skills of leadership are not easily acquired or generally well taught. Good leaders do not make all the decisions themselves and then tell others what to do! They recognize that the skill and knowledge contained in the team is far wider and deeper than that of any individual member (including the leader) and seek to create a climate in which those skills and that knowledge can be fully used in the provision and development of services (13, 14).

Team building and maintenance are essential activities if the most effective and efficient pattern of multi-disciplinary working is to be achieved. Shared accommodation, democracy over who makes the coffee and who does the washing up, informal chats over lunch and more formal team-development meetings are all important.

10.6 EDUCATIONAL ACTIVITY

We make no apology for mentioning this in a 'practical' textbook. Education is a primary activity for all psychogeriatric teams. In many centres, this will include the undergraduate and postgraduate training of doctors, nurses and other professional groups within the health service. It will also include offering help in training social services staff and working with voluntary bodies in providing input into carers groups and staff training. More than that, it involves viewing each contact with patient or carer as an opportunity for education. A third to a half of consultation time may be spent explaining to patient (and carer) the nature of the health problem they appear to have and possible ways of managing this, always encouraging and listening for feedback, so that the management plan is acceptable to patient and carer.

In educating students, we aim to improve their **knowledge**, develop their **skills** and (sometimes) change their **attitudes**. Knowledge is acquired through lectures, reading, seminars, etc. Generally, the more 'processing' someone has to do with their knowledge, the better it is understood and consolidated. Skills are acquired by supervised practice, and attitudes are changed by exposure to people with different attitudes in favourable circumstances. There is evidence that a good course in health care of the elderly can improve medical students attitudes as well as their knowledge [15].

10.7 RESEARCH AND DEVELOPMENT

Research is sometimes thought of as a rather esoteric activity. However, it can be a very practical approach to analysing what services are needed and how they are delivered. The systematic evaluation of alternative patterns of care has always been a weakness in health and social services' provision, and deserves more attention from professional bodies and journals. We tend rather to provide services that seem a 'good idea' (if they are not too expensive). Some developments such as 'care planning' and 'case management' are implemented without researching and providing the resources to ensure their success.

At an even simpler level, hospital doctors can find out what information GPs value in letters about patients and whether patients prefer to be seen at home or in the clinic.

Components of complicated services can be analysed to see whether there are better ways of achieving the same objectives. This, for example, has recently been done with respect to domiciliary versus day-hospital physiotherapy for post-stroke patients [16] and for intensive day-hospital versus inpatient care for younger psychiatric inpatients [17]. We do not all have the resources or time to develop major research projects of the kind that are published in medical journals, but we all can adopt a progressive and open-minded approach to finding out what people want from our services (as well as what they **need**) and developing those services. This is particularly important at a time when health-care systems in many countries are coming under financial and political pressure to deliver 'value for money'. Perhaps the motto 'there may be a better way' should be tattooed on all our foreheads!

10.8 AUDIT AND QUALITY

Another facet of the changes in health services in the UK has been a more self-conscious attitude to audit and quality. If research tells us the best treatments to use, audit tells us whether we are delivering them effectively. Medical audit is essentially a method of education and quality improvement. In our service, the medical staff take one afternoon a month to meet together and audit some aspect of our service. We look at issues like the prescribing of anti-depressants, the assessment of dementia, the use of day hospital, communication on patient discharge and seek to agree standards against which we then audit our practice. Such audits sometimes reveal that we do not do things as we think they should be done, and repeat audits can then check whether standards are improving. Some people would argue that without this 'audit cycle' no true audit is being done. There is, however, a danger of bureaucratizing the process of quality management and trying to agree detailed procedures for everything which are then monitored from the top down. This approach is worse than useless since it creates an 'us and them' attitude and does not value the integrity of the individual worker. Management do need indicators that quality is being pursued but they do not need to be involved in every detail of the process. Audit is also carried out in other disciplines and increasingly in a multi-disciplinary setting.

10.9 BUSINESS PLANNING

Planning in the National Health Service used to be in large committees on which practitioners were variably represented. Joint planning with social services involved even larger committees where most members (especially from the social services' side) had no contact with service users. Now provider units and trusts have adopted an industrial model of business planning where there is more involvement of the 'coal-face' workers. We are encouraged to use the techniques of 'SWOT' (Strengths, Weaknesses, Opportunities and Threats) analysis to produce annual development plans. It is an invigorating process but a problem persists in trying to develop this approach within the quasi-market since success does not always bring extra funds in the same way it might in a less complicated real market. Nevertheless, a 'bottom-up' approach to planning is much to be preferred to one that is exclusively 'top-down'. The wider issues of the health needs of the population are now to be addressed by the purchasers of health care, the district health authorities and fund-holding GPs conducting 'needs' assessments' for their populations and purchasing services accordingly. This is certainly an exciting departure from previous cooperative systems of planning and has led to rapidly increasing management costs (up 900 per cent nationally) without any clear overall change in health-service delivery, so far. One danger is that the expertise of clinicians in the area of needs assessment may be neglected because they have been identified with the 'providers' rather than the 'purchasers' of health care. The new structure also puts a premium on negotiating skills which clinicians may need to develop [18].

10.10 LEGAL ASPECTS

10.10.1 Different approaches

American and United Kingdom law and practice in relation to mental health and compulsory treatment show interesting differences. United Kingdom law is encapsulated in the Mental Health Act (1983) which has been explored in some detail by Bluglass [19]. Two strands can be detected in both United Kingdom and American legislation. The first is the necessity to protect others from someone else's madness. This has been described as a sort of 'policing' function. The second is the need to protect the interests of the mentally ill person against exploitation and to ensure that people with severe mental illness receive appropriate treatment sometimes even when they do not see their need for this. This can be described as a kind of 'parental' function. In England and Wales, the Vagrancy Acts of 1713 and 1744 allowed the detention of people with mental illness who might be dangerous on the order of two or more justices and the Madhouses Act of 1744 tried to ensure minimum standards in private institutions. Thus the two strands of legislation can be seen even at that early date. The Mental Health Act (1959) firmly moved the care of people who were mentally disordered away from the judicial into the medical sphere (except when a crime had been committed). This tradition has been maintained in the Mental Health Act (1983) though Mental Health Review Tribunals of a quasi-judicial nature have been introduced to give patients a right of appeal against their detention. In the UK the question of patients' capability to handle their own affairs is dealt with quite separately from the question of detention and compulsory treatment under the somewhat archaic institution of the Court of Protection. In the USA where litigation and lawyers are more frequently encountered than in the UK, judicial procedures have been retained although 'competency' and 'commitment' hearings are no longer linked. Each state has its own mental health code. Some states even have a 'bill of rights' for inpatients including a 'right' to the best quality of care.

10.10.2 'Inspection'

The presence of a legal framework does not of itself ensure quality of care, and audit and quality management are seen as increasingly important in many health-care systems. In addition, the UK system deals with these issues through the Health Advisory Service, a sort of benign national inspectorate, and the Mental Health Commission of the 1983 Act. American legislation appears to be going through many changes and the section on the law in *A Comprehensive Textbook of Psychiatry* [20] questions whether the trend in the USA to medicalize deviant behaviour is now being replaced by a tendency to criminalize mentally ill people.

10.10.3 Consent and the law

United Kingdom and American law also differ in their interpretation of the question of consent to treatment. In the USA 'informed' consent is the term used to cover the patient's right to know all about the likely effects and risks of treatment. The UK legal concept of consent ('real' consent) allows the doctor discretion to decide exactly how much information to give to the patent; the doctor still has a duty to inform the patient but the extent of this information is to be judged by what would be regarded as good medical practice and not by some absolute duty to disclose everything. A useful recent document on consent and the incapacitated adult by the Law Commission reviews the law in the United Kingdom and other jurisdictions (21).

10.10.4 The Mental Health Act (1983)

The remainder of this discussion will be devoted to legislation in England and Wales. The **Mental Health Act** of 1983 has sections that deal with compulsory admission for assessment (Section 2, Section 4 in emergency) and for treatment (Section 3) as well as enabling a voluntary patient who is already receiving treatment to be detained in hospital (Section 5) for up to 72 hours to enable a Section 2 or Section 3 to be implemented.

(a) Section 2

Section 2 is the standard means of compelling a patient to go into hospital for up to 28 days' assessment (which can include necessary treatment). An application must be made by an approved social worker or the patient's (legally defined) nearest relative. Two medical recommendations are necessary, one normally from a doctor who has known the patient for some time (usually the General Practitioner), the other from a doctor approved by the Secretary of State for Health under Section 12 of the Mental Health Act as having special experience in the diagnosis and treatment of mental disorders (usually a consultant or senior registrar in psychiatry). In their recommendations the doctors must state that the patient is suffering from mental disorder of a nature or degree that warrants detention in hospital and that compulsory admission is necessary in the interests of the patient's health or safety or for the protection of others. The patient and his or her nearest relative, when possible, must be informed of the implementation of the Section and of rights of appeal. There are carefully defined rights of appeal to specially set up Mental Health Review Tribunals and the hospital managers also have the ability to discharge a patient. The responsible consultant or the nearest relative may discharge the patient from the Section at any time but the responsible doctor can block the relative's right of discharge under certain circumstances. Once the papers have been completed, the social worker has the right to take steps to convey the patient to a hospital which has agreed to accept him. A representative of hospital managers (usually a senior nurse) must formally receive the patient and the papers.

(b) Section 4

Section 4 depends on an application and the medical recommendation of only one doctor. It is only to be used in an emergency if undue delay would result from seeking a second opinion. The use of this Section has to be justified and explained on the relevant legal document. It lasts for only 72 hours, otherwise in most respects it is similar to Section 2.

(c) Section 3

Section 3 is a treatment Section (although necessary treatment may also be given under Section 2). It again requires two medical recommendations although they must be more detailed in this case. The application can be made by a social worker but in this case the nearest relative's consent is essential. Exceptionally, the nearest relative can be displaced by legal action. Section 3 lasts initially for six months. The nearest relative, as well as the responsible medical officer, has the right of discharge although again the relative's right can be blocked in certain circumstances by the responsible medical officer. The patient must be informed of his rights including rights of appeal. A particular line of treatment cannot be continued beyond three months without the patient's consent or the support of a second opinion from a designated doctor.

Specific treatments (presently only psychosurgery and the surgical implantation of hormones) can only be given with the patient's consent **and** the approval of a Mental Health Tribunal. Other treatment (for example, ECT) can only be given with the patient's consent or, under Section 3, with a second opinion from a designated doctor.

(d) Section 5(2)

Section 5(2) enables the responsible medical officer or a named deputy to detain a previously voluntary inpatient for up to 72 hours while a Section 2 or Section 3 is implemented. Section 5(4) is a holding power for designated senior nurses which can only be implemented if a patient is already receiving inpatient treatment for mental disorder, only extends for six hours and is only used when it is not practicable to secure the immediate attendance of a medical practitioner to implement Section 5(2).

(e) Guardianship under Section 7 of the Mental Health Act

This confers upon the guardian the power to require the patient to reside at a specified place, to attend for treatment (widely defined) and to require access to the patient at any place where they may be residing for a doctor, approved social worker or other person. Guardianship orders can only be applied to people over the age of 16 years and need the consent of the nearest relative, an application from an approved social worker (or the nearest relative) and two medical recommendations. The local social services authority has to agree to accept the guardianship order and to approve the guardian if he or she is not a member of the social services staff. Perhaps because guardianship orders are essentially difficult to enforce without the co-operation of the patient, they are not used nearly so frequently as other Mental Health Act Sections (just over 120 in England and Wales each year compared with an annual rate of 15 000 compulsory admissions [22]). However, when they are used, it is predominantly in old people, to enable them to be looked after in their own homes or, more often, in residential care [22, 23].

(f) Court orders

Other parts of the Mental Health Act enable the courts to remand patients to hospital for report on their mental condition, to remand them to hospital for treatment and to make interim hospital orders so that the offender's response in hospital can be evaluated without irrevocable commitment to this method of dealing with the offender if it should prove unsuitable. There is also a court equivalent of the Section 7 guardianship power. These court powers are rarely used with old people and will not be discussed in any detail here.

(g) The mental health legislation and the demented patient

When is detention detention? The common-law duty of care means that, when looking after confused patients, staff have to take reasonable precautions against them wandering off and coming into danger. A 'confusion lock' (usually a door with two handles, both of which have to be operated simultaneously, or a combination lock with the number displayed near it) is as big an obstacle to some (though not all!) demented patients as a mortice lock to a mentally well person. It would, however, be extremely cumbersome, restrictive and expensive to put all demented inpatients on Section 2 or Section 3 and would be against the spirit of successive Mental Health Acts which have sought to reduce the need for compulsory detention. Most doctors prefer to treat their demented patients informally except under exceptional circumstances. Nurse staffing levels can be highly relevant here, as informal care is often possible with an adequate number of nurses whereas a shortage of nurses is more likely to lead to the need for locked doors.

Many demented patients in hospital do not understand where they are and, almost by definition, they are unable to understand treatment or give fully informed consent in the same way that a person who was mentally well or, indeed, suffering from another form of mental illness might. It is considered essential under the Mental Health Act that formally detained patients who cannot give consent should have their treatment reviewed at three months by a doctor designated to do this work by the Mental Health Act Commission. Should not the same standard also apply to informal patients with dementia who are not able fully to understand their treatment? This is a difficult question. Its answer hinges on the interpretation of 'consent'. UK law has so far taken the view that the doctor can exercise professional judgement in deciding how much information should be given to a patient in seeking to obtain consent, and has adhered to the concept of 'real' consent (see above). The potential expense and bureaucracy of over-eager application of the Mental Health Act is enormous and health professionals, especially doctors and social workers, have to perform a delicate balancing act between their patients' 'right to consent' and what is reasonable and in patients' best interests.

10.10.5 The Court of Protection and power of attorney

An 'enduring' or 'deferred' power of attorney is now available in England and Wales as it is in Scotland and some other countries. This enables a person when mentally capable of understanding their affairs and the nature and effect of a power of attorney, to provide for someone else to manage their affairs if they became incapable. The power becomes effective when registered with the Court of Protection. The only alternative for management of a demented patient's affairs is the

Court of Protection which can be unduly cumbersome and expensive, especially if only small amounts of money are involved. Application to the Court is usually made through a solicitor and may be made by a relative, solicitor or doctor or other interested person. Usually the application is made by a near relative of the patient. The Court requires a medical report and serves notice on the patient, through his doctor, that a 'hearing' will be held at a specified time and place. Following this hearing, a receiver is appointed to look after the patient's affairs under the supervision of the Court. The Court was originally set up to manage a relatively small number of cases and is in danger of being swamped by the volume of work with the increasing number of demented old people. However, there are moves to introduce new laws on the issues of consent and the incapacitated adult. In the meantime, many relatives exercise financial control over the affairs of demented patients in a less formal way (for example, through authorities to draw cheques on the patient's bank account). These authorities have often, though not always, been issued early in the course of the patient's illness when they were able to make some judgement about such matters, and relatives do not always appreciate that they may be no longer valid when the patient becomes incapacitated. Although the legal status of such powers is dubious and they cannot be recommended, in many cases they do seem to work!

10.11 CONCLUSION

The emphasis of this book has been on the practice rather than the theory of psychiatry with old people. We have tried to cover these practical aspects thoroughly and to give appropriate references for those who wish to pursue them. Our aim has been to show that the proper psychiatric care of mentally ill old people is immensely worthwhile and rewarding. We have pointed to political and managerial issues as well as purely psychiatric issues as we believe that proper care for old people is dependent upon the political, managerial and economic commitment to provide it. We hope that you have found the book useful and thought-provoking and that you have enjoyed reading it as much as we have enjoyed writing it.

REFERENCES

1. Royal College of Psychiatrists (1987) Guidelines for regional advisers on consultant posts in the psychiatry of old age. *Bulletin of the Royal College of Psychiatrists*, **11**, 240–2.
2. Royal College of Psychiatrists (1992) *The Mental Health of the Nation: the Contribution of Psychiatrists*, Royal College of Psychiatrists, London.
3. Snowdon, J. (1991) Bed requirements for an area psychogeriatric service. *Australian and New Zealand Journal of Psychiatry*, **25**, 56–62.
4. Wattis, J.P. (1988) Geographical variations in the provision of psychiatric services for old people. *Age and Ageing*, **17**, 171–80.
5. Department of Health and Social Security (1972) *Services for Mental Illness Related to Old Age*, HM(72)71, DHSS, London.
6. National Health Service, Health Advisory Service (1982) *The Rising Tide: Developing Services for Mental Illness in Old Age*, NHS Health Advisory Service, Sutton, Surrey.
7. The Royal College of Physicians of London and The Royal College of Psychiatrists (1989) *Care of Elderly People with Mental Illness: Specialist Services and Medical Training*, Royal College of Physicians and Royal College of Psychiatrists, London.
8. Wattis, J.P., Hobson, J. and Barker, G. (1992) Needs for continuing care of demented people: a model for estimating needs. *Psychiatric Bulletin*, **16**, 465–7.
9. Centre for Policy on Ageing (1984) *Home Life: a Code of Practice for Residential Care*, CPA, London.
10. Kitwood, T. and Bredin, K. (1992) A new approach to the evaluation of dementia care. *Journal of Advances in Health and Nursing Care*, **1**(5), 41–60.
11. Libow, L.S., Schechter, Z. and Margolis, E. (1981) Demographic and economic aspects, in *The Core of Geriatric Medicine*, (eds L.S. Libow and F.T. Sherman), The Mosby Company, St Louis, Missouri.
12. Department of Health (1990) Joint Health/Social Services Circular: Health and Social Services Development: *'Caring for People', the Care Programme Approach for People with a Mental Illness Referred to the Specialist Psychiatric Services*, HC(90)23/LASSL(90)11, Department of Health Publications Unit, London.
13. Harvey-Jones, J. (1989) *Making it Happen: Reflections on Leadership*, Fontana, London.
14. Wattis, J.P. (1987) Working with other disciplines, in *A Handbook for Trainee Psychiatrists*, (ed. K.J. Rix), Baillière Tindall, London.
15. Smith, C.W. and Wattis, J.P. (1989) Medical students' attitudes to old people and career preference: the case of Nottingham Medical School. *Medical Education*, **23**, 81–5.
16. Young, J. and Forster, A. (1992) The Bradford community stroke trial: results at six months. *British Medical Journal*, **304**, 1085–9.
17. Creed, F., Black, D. and Anthony, P. (1989) Day hospital and com-

munity treatment for acute psychiatric illness: a critical appraisal. *British Journal of Psychiatry*, **154**, 300–10.

18. Kennedy, G., Benson, J. and McMillan, J. (1991) *Managing Negotiations*, Business Books Ltd., London.
19. Bluglass, R. (1984) *A Guide to the Mental Health Act*, Churchill Livingstone, London.
20. Kaplan, H.I. and Sadock, B. (1985) *A Comprehensive Textbook of Psychiatry*, Williams & Williams, Baltimore.
21. The Law Commission (1991) *Mentally Incapacitated Adults and Decision Making: an Overview*, Consultation Paper Number 119, HMSO, London.
22. Grant, W. (1992) Guardianship orders: a review of their use under the 1983 Mental Health Act. *Medicine, Science and the Law*, **32**, 319–24.
23. Wattis, J.P., Grant, W., Traynor, J. and Harris, S. (1990) Use of guardianship under the 1983 Mental Health Act. *Medicine, Science and the Law*, **30**, 313–16.

Index

Page numbers appearing in **bold** refer to figures and page numbers appearing in *italic* refer to tables.